FEEL GOOD,
LOOK GOOD,
FOR LIFE

Barbra,

Believe it can be! *

♡ Angela

ISBN: 978-0-9979801-4-1
Published in 2016 by Blue Star Publishing

Cover design by Paul Vorreiter
Interior design by Michelle M. White
Graphics design by Michelle M. White
Author photos by Eric Weber
Editorial review by Alexandra O'Connell

Printed in the United States of America
First Edition

www.AngelaGaffney.com

FEEL GOOD, LOOK GOOD, FOR LIFE

Your Ultimate Guide to Achieve Lifelong Health

Angela Gaffney

BLUE STAR
PUBLISHING

To Rob, Tori and Sean

You are my shining stars.

Contents

Introduction

"Mrs. Gaffney, we have good news and bad news to share with you today," my doctor said. "The good news is that we know what's going on in your body. You have a rare neuromuscular disease called Mitochondrial Myopathy. The bad news is that it's a progressive disease; it will attack your various organ systems and cause drooping eyelids, diabetes, blindness, deafness and paralysis.

"I've never heard of a positive outcome. You need to go home, read as much literature as you can and prepare for what's to come."

The pit in my stomach grew larger and larger as each word left his mouth. My heart fell deep into the ground beneath my feet; I was in shock. I thought this was supposed to be the new beginning, the day I would receive my answer and figure out a plan to repair my broken body.

It felt like my life fell apart in an instant, but the reality was it had taken years for this unruly, inexplicable event to occur. I had plenty of thoughts through the years about how my life might pan out and never in my wildest dreams did I expect to be told I needed to go home to prepare for a disease to progressively attack my body, and in the end, take my life. There were many dark days to follow this news, but in time my journey would include days of positive movement forward, each bringing me one step closer to regaining my health. I wish the same for you, and this is why I've written this book.

My biggest hope is that you learn new ways to make health happen in your life, simply because you, my friend, deserve it! One big lesson I've learned throughout my journey is that my choices at the table and in life feed me in health and happiness. I contributed to my ill body, and the dis-ease that was taking place. It is impossible to change everything overnight, but you can take one simple step each and every day to move forward, make a difference in your health and happiness, and transform your life. It is my belief that the body has the ability to heal itself when given the right tools and a lot of love. If you're ready to begin your journey, I would be thrilled to support you along the way!

Each section of this book shares part of my personal journey, and provides you with tools that will challenge your thoughts, help you create new habits, learn new behaviors, and forever change your life. I'll give you fair warning that it's not a piece of cake, and there'll be bumps along the road so I'll help guide you during these difficult times too. This book is your guide to feel good and look good for life; but it is only that. A guide. The magic comes when you implement everything I share with you. You'll need to complete the exercises, practice the strategies, build awareness, and choose differently in order to create change in your life. Health is possible for each and every one of us, and I'm excited to be on this journey with you!

There are a few key rules you must abide by while making health happen:

- To yourself you must be true; take responsibility for all you do.
- Be open to new possibilities, ideas and thoughts.
- Respect all the emotions that surface during your journey.
- Release the need to control the responses of others.
- Above all, always be kind to YOU.

It's time for healthy transformation. Let's explore the strategies, stories and exercises that will help you feel good and look good for life!

SECTION I

Your #1 Fan is Looking for Love

We hustle through life at such a quick pace that we often forget the one who supports us the most. I know you have a lot of fans cheering you on in life, but these aren't the people I'm speaking of. I'm talking about the one who shows up for you every single day, no matter the situation, and supports you beyond measure.

Your #1 fan and greatest supporter in this life is your body!

It wasn't until my body was failing beyond measure that I realized that I needed to have a healthy relationship with it. Never once did I consider that my body might actually need a little support and care from me. I woke up every day knowing it'd be there to carry me through. Until the day it didn't. This first section of the book will help you build a healthy relationship with your #1 fan. Take the time you need to explore the exercises, gain awareness, and practice the strategies I provide you. It's time to give your #1 fan the love it's looking for.

CHAPTER 1

I'm Not Sick, But I'm Not Well

At what point do we stop and say, "I can feel better than this?"

It took me quite a while to realize that I could feel better, and function at a higher level than I was used to. I went undiagnosed for almost two years while my body continued to deteriorate. Severe joint pain and inflammation, chronic stomach aches, brain fog, and very weak muscles were now a part of me. During that time I lost my ability to write because I could no longer hold a pen, simple daily tasks of brushing my teeth and combing my hair meant I had to work through severe pain, and my energy was so low that I functioned for about 20 minutes out of a 10 hour day. It wasn't until months after I was diagnosed that I started to explore the idea that I could feel better, and work with this idea that my body had the ability to heal.

I Can Feel Better Than This

I meet people every day who generally don't feel good. They are dealing with autoimmune disease, obesity, fatigue, pain, and more, and for the most part they can't see any way out of it. I too felt this way; when I was in the thick of it I couldn't see beyond my symptoms, and the fear of losing the high-functioning life I knew consumed me. But the great news is that I was able to find a way out, and so can you!

The book is divided into three sections for you:

1. Your #1 Fan is Looking for Love
2. Building a Solid Foundation
3. The Care and Keeping of You

Each section has a theme: the first focuses on self-care, the second section will help you build a foundation for long-term health, and the final section provides guidance to nurture yourself through the process. This layout will provide you the opportunity to:

- Explore the choices you make in your life today;
- Understand how you can enhance your health through life food and table food;
- Learn how to build a healthy foundation; beginning with whole food nourishment;
- Decide how you want to participate in your life going forward;
- Set yourself up for long-term success.

Many areas of life affect our health; it's not just about dieting. That's why this book flips dieting on its head. We're going to focus on what's most important to achieve long-term health: nourishing your body in every aspect of life. That's why Section I begins with information that might not immediately appear to be food-related. My goal is for you to feel good and look good for life, and that includes and goes beyond the food we eat.

The best way to use this book is to read through each chapter, take time to complete the exercises I share with you and revisit different chapters and sections of the book when you need a quick review or have a question. Each chapter is outlined for you in the Table of Contents for quick reference and ease. I've also shared a few recipes in the book, so enjoy the wonderful flavors and nourishment.

The end of the book contains a section for additional resources so you may continue to grow your health knowledge, explore new ideas and research, and identify ways to support yourself in health and happiness. You may also visit me at www.AngelaGaffney.com for more information and to connect directly if you have any questions; I'd love to hear from you.

We get used to functioning at whatever level the body functions at; people are used to feeling tired every morning, experience an afternoon lull or headache most days of the week. They live with aching joints, and some experience tummy aches all the time. But what if there was a way to change all of this? What if there were simple steps you could take that would change the way you think about health, empower you to make healthy choices without restriction and guilt, and in the end transform your life? What would you do with this opportunity?

It's time to find out . . .

Here's the first exercise of many that you'll explore while reading this book; all in the name of creating the healthiest, happiest life you can imagine.

EXERCISE: *Letter to Your Body*

I encourage you to write this letter as if you're writing to a dear friend. Share all that you wish for, all that you may be sorry for, and also share your goals, and how you plan to support your body in this journey. It's a time for reflection, and clarity. Most often, we have a challenging relationship with our body; always wanting more from it, being critical of its form, and wishing our wrinkles away. This causes a lot of grief, and with a struggling relationship such as this, we tend to rebel, show little respect, and demand that the body show up for us no matter what we put it through. This hits home for me, as I remember the days when my relationship with my body was a battle, instead of a relationship of love and gratitude as it is today. Health begins with this one step. Take time to sit quietly and express everything you'd like to share with this dear body of yours; it's supported you through thick and thin and will do so for all your days. What would you like to say to it in return?

When you write your letter please consider the following: How have you treated your body? Is there anything you wished you would have done differently? You may even feel the need to apologize, and that is fine too. This is an opportunity for you to consider past habits and choices, share how you'd like to work together in the days to come, and achieve your health goals while building a strong relationship. This is an important exercise, so grab your pen or pencil, find a quiet space and start writing! We'll revisit this letter later in the book, and having done this will provide you:

- *A new perspective into this relationship*
- *A baseline for setting health goals*
- *A way to track progress as you journey through this book and into life*

To My Amazing Body,

Love,

Congratulations; you've taken a powerful step to creating health and happiness in your life! Cherish the words you've shared in this letter. Move forward without judgement, but rather knowing you and your body have what it takes to work together to achieve your goals. You're an amazing team.

I'm Not Sick, But I'm Not Well

I encounter many people who believe that pain, weight gain, fatigue and chronic headaches are all just "a part of getting older." All too often, life is accompanied by high blood pressure, high cholesterol, diabetes and excess weight, chronic pain, fatigue and headaches. Rarely does anyone, including me at one point, choose to dig deep and understand how their choices in life contribute to their ailing body.

It's time we step up to the plate, investigate the reasons behind our health ailments and realize that it's not just a part of growing old. We all hope that life is for a very long time, but we should desire to have our quality of life for the long haul too. If we don't do the work now, that won't exist.

There are two areas to consider when creating health for the long haul: Life Food and Table Food. Our environment includes our relationships, our work, our home life, and more…all of these areas, our "Life Food," need to be addressed just as much as our "Table Food" environment which includes everything we put into our body. You'll be empowered to explore both of these areas as you navigate through this book, and it is my hope that it'll inspire you to love life, feel vibrant and be healthy!

Life Food and Table Food

This book is full of exercises to help you explore your health needs, identify areas of strength and growth, and implement the Life Food and Table Food tips I share with you.

Each Life Food exercise will be tagged with this symbol:

Each Table Food exercise will be tagged with this symbol:

Remember that Table Food refers to the food we eat to nourish our body; whole grains, leafy greens, fruits, vegetables and more. We'll be discussing the quality of the food we nourish our body with a lot, and it'll be important for you to consider the choices you're making today, and your personal goals moving forward.

Life Food includes everything outside of the food and drink we consume as fuel. It includes our relationships, finances, spirituality and faith, volunteerism, exercise, connection with nature and more. It will help you consider the choices you're making in life, and identify whether your choices are increasing fulfillment, or perhaps negating it. Health happens when we nourish the body in both areas of Table Food and Life Food; we can't perform at our best if one area is out of alignment with our values and goals. Lucky for you, this book will help you grow in each area, and achieve optimal health and happiness.

I'm not sick, but I'm not well. There are so many people functioning at a less-than-optimal level that it's become the norm to live in survival mode. But why couldn't everyone thrive instead?

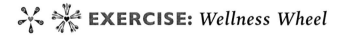 EXERCISE: *Wellness Wheel*

It's time to dive into life. This wheel consists of 15 different areas that all feed into your health and happiness. The goal is to see where your wheel is adequately "filled" versus areas where you may be a little flat.

Before you begin the exercise, though, I want to provide some differentiation between two key words: success and fulfillment.

This exercise is focused on the fulfillment in your life versus your success in life. Here's the difference: fulfillment is defined as the "satisfaction or happiness as a result of fully developing one's abilities or character" or "the achievement of something desired, promised, or predicted." Success, rather, only focuses on the accomplishment of an aim or purpose; it has nothing to do with the happiness or joy you feel as a result of developing your abilities or character. There's a big difference, folks; you can achieve your career goals, even climb the corporate ladder all the way to the top, but if you wake up every morning stressed and hating your job, you have achieved success but are void of fulfillment. On the other hand, you could land the job you've always wanted (success) and love going into work every day because you experience so much joy and happiness as a result (fulfillment) and have the best of both worlds. In this case, you've achieved success and fulfillment at the same time!

This wheel is only concerned with your fulfillment; the satisfaction or happiness you feel as a result of fully developing your abilities or character.

The wheel has a spoke for each life area, a heart in the center, and a bold outer circle line. Assess one life area at a time, considering how FULFILLED you are in this area, and do the following:

- *If you're completely fulfilled in this area you will place a dot where the line meets the outer circle.*
- *If you are completely unfulfilled, you will place a dot where the line meets the center heart.*

- *If you're like most of us, you may not be completely fulfilled in all areas of life; in this case you'll want to place your dot anywhere on the line in between the heart (unfulfilled) and outer circle (completely fulfilled) to identify your level of fulfillment in that area of life.*
- *Once you've placed all your dots in the wheel, connect the dots to see the shape of your wheel.*

Wellness Wheel

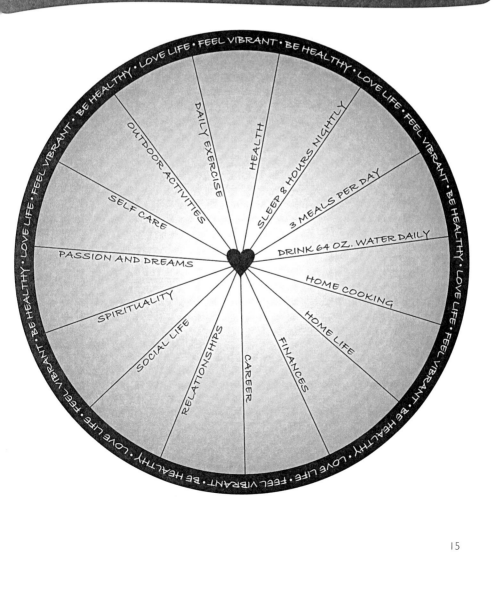

How's Your Wellness Wheel Rolling?

Don't be alarmed if your wheel is flat in areas, pointed in others, and nicely rounded in spots. The wheel will look different depending on life circumstances, our health, and overall happiness. The best part of this exercise is that it provides us the big picture of our life; it offers an opportunity to focus on key areas and increase fulfillment. This exercise should be completed every 3-6 months to assess growth, readjust, and decide what your next focus will be. I often suggest that you create a "key" for your entries, using a different colored pen to complete your wheel exercise each time, and logging a date in the upper right hand corner of your page with the same colored ink pen to log your entries.

When this exercise is complete, I'd like you to select one or two areas you'd like to focus on and enter them into your personal notes below.

Personal Notes

The two areas I'd like to focus on to achieve increased fulfillment are:

    1._____

    2._____

One thing I can do to increase fulfillment in each of these areas is:

    1._____

    2._____

Keep these life areas in mind as you work through this book; you'll be provided strategies to support you in personal growth and fulfillment as you continue the journey toward feeling good, and looking good, for life.

CHAPTER 2

Building Awareness

W hat has your body told you today? Were you tired when you woke up, maybe have the sniffles, or experience a headache? Our bodies speak to us all day long but most often we don't take the time to listen or, furthermore, respond.

Listen to Your Body. It Always Tells the Truth

I spent the first 35 years of my life depending on this body of mine to carry me through whatever I wanted to do. Never once did I recognize the need to check in with my body and understand what it might need from me. There was plenty of talking going on long before my symptoms aggressively attacked, but I took these little whispers as annoyances. I'd pop a few Motrin when my joints were acting up, depend on caffeine when my fatigue was setting in, and truly thought that it'd all just pass. Eventually, the messages got louder and louder, until my body was literally screaming at me. If I had responded to the whispers early on, my journey might not have been so difficult.

The body always tell the truth. It's a beautifully connected system and when all parts are working properly, we function at a high level. Living with fatigue, pain, digestive issues and more aren't "normal" and they certainly are not a part of the "aging" process. Stop with any excuse you may be giving yourself and start digging into the issue at hand. When you become aware of the symptoms you're experiencing, you can explore ways to turn things around and achieve health.

Each symptom that occurs in the body has a root cause. More times than not, our diet and life choices directly impact the cause of our symptoms. Start taking note of your symptoms, understand that this is the body's way of speaking to you, and most importantly stay positive in the thought that our bodies were created to heal when provided love and the correct tools.

The choices you make in life and the food you eat directly impact the needs of your body. Once you are aware of the symptoms you may be experiencing, start taking a peek into the choices you're making around table food and life food. Are these choices supportive of your body, or stressing it out? If you find choices that are stressing the body, then it's time to dig deeper and uncover why you make the choices you do.

Prior to my health crisis, I lived on sugar and Diet Coke. It was of course all low-fat as well as low-calorie and I thought I was doing very well for myself. I was very active and fit and had no clue my internal health was struggling. In the beginning of my ill days I would wish away the heart palpitations, headaches, fatigue, digestive issues, and pain. I never thought for a moment that I was contributing to every bit of the failure taking place.

I was wrong.

Just as a good friend would alert you to a problem, the body does the same. Too often we push these little messages under the rug, and sometimes even get upset when our body doesn't function like we think it should. It's time to be thankful for the communication, and understand that the body has an amazing ability to fight, and heal, and live well; it sometimes just needs a little extra attention and TLC to get the job done.

It's time to check in with your own body, and take a listen to what it's telling you. Remember that sometimes it's a whisper, a sniffle or small ache, and other times it's screaming a message loud and clear. Be respectful of however your body is speaking to you and log your inventory in the exercise below:

❊ EXERCISE: *My Body Inventory*

Please circle or highlight any symptoms, big or small, that your body is expressing. I have provided you a list of ideas to work from, but it is not all inclusive. Please add any additional symptoms you may be feeling in the inventory log.

Symptoms:
- Fatigue
- Headaches
- Migraines
- Brain fog
- Dizziness
- Congestion
- Digestive problems
- Heart burn
- Bloating
- Gas
- Constipation
- Diarrhea
- Dry skin

- Brittle nails
- White coating on tongue
- Joint pain
- Muscle pain
- Weight gain
- Obesity
- Diabetes
- Heart disease
- Auto-immune disease (Crohn's, arthritis, psoriasis, etc.)
- High blood pressure
- High cholesterol (LDL, triglycerides)
- Repressed immune system (often get colds, bronchitis, flu, strep throat)

My body speaks to me by expressing these symptoms:

_____

_____

_____

_____

_____

_____

_____

_____

My Body Inventory: ADDITIONAL SYMPTOMS

_____

_____

_____

_____

_____

_____

_____

_____

_____

_____

I would like to take the following steps to explore the cause of my ailing body:

1._____

2._____

3._____

Finding the Good!

Have you ever been in such a deep hole that you couldn't see even a flicker of light? In the depths of my illness, I never once considered that anything good could come of my situation. In the end, though, I realized the struggle was one of the greatest gifts I could've been given in this lifetime. Can you think of a similar situation in your own life?

We don't always understand why things happen, or the timing of an occurrence or event. What I've come to learn is that our lives are beautifully designed, and perfect in their own right. This doesn't mean that everything goes just as we'd like it to, or happen just as we would expect. However, with each life circumstance we have the opportunity to learn something about ourselves. This has been one of the best parts of my journey back to health. An amazing mentor of mine once said that the frustrations I may have with others are there to help me take a look at my own areas for improvement. I had shared an example with her of my husband being short with me during a conversation. I felt like he was distracted, looking at his phone and not truly listening to what I had to say. When I took a step back and turned this frustration on myself, I asked, "How was I short in this situation? Could I have listened better? Was I distracted?"

The answer was yes, I was definitely being short with my words and I was not the most patient person during the conversation. The most insightful part of this exercise though was the listening question. "Could I have listened better?" While I was caught up in wondering if I could have listened better to him, I realized that the bigger problem was that I wasn't listening to myself! I had asked his opinion about something that he really didn't care about and I saw him disengage. All along, the answer was right inside of me; I just wasn't choosing to listen.

Many of you may relate when I say I love seeking input and asking others what they think about "stuff"...business stuff, mom stuff, fashion stuff, exercise stuff...you name it. I enjoy getting input from others on just about everything. While it's okay to ask the input of others, we must keep in mind that the answers to most, if not all that we need to know when making decisions for ourselves, are right inside of us. We tend to ask others their thoughts and opinions for our own validation, instead of moving forward with what we know is true and best for ourselves. It is our job to trust the answers that reside within us, and with confidence move forward.

There is good in everything. In the small moments that provide us self-reflection and opportunity to grow as well as the big moments when life-shattering experiences stop us in our tracks and forever change our lives. What good do you need to explore? What frustrations are there to help you look inside yourself and create healthy change?

✳ EXERCISE: *Finding the Good*

What is your biggest challenge with seeing the good, and trusting that it's there in all circumstances?

_____

_____

_____

_____

_____

_____

_____

_____

How does goodness exist in your own life?

_____

_____

_____

_____

_____

_____

Please write about a challenging experience that brought goodness into your life.
- *How long did it take for you to be able to see the good?*
- *How have you learned from the experience?*
- *Has anything changed for you as a result of this experience; spirituality, belief in others, etc.?*

_____

_____

_____
_____
_____
_____
_____
_____
_____
_____
_____
_____
_____
_____
_____
_____
_____
_____
_____
_____
_____
_____
_____

Forgive Yourself for the Not-So-Great Moments

My daughter was in third grade when this "mom-of-the-year" event took place...

Tori's turn for "student of the month" came around late in the school year. She happily brought the poster home to color and log information about her favorite foods, places she'd visited, and more. She had worked on it for days, and I was so proud of the work she put into it. One evening, she was home with the sitter and finished up her project. The kids were in bed when I returned home so the following morning she proudly shared her poster with me...the poster that'd be hanging up in school to celebrate the beautiful child she is. This is what I read in the "Likes" and "Dislikes" area of the poster: "Dislikes": Spinach and my mom yelling all the time. What?!?!?! The only thing I could think was *Wow, I made the poster!*

"Tori," I said, "Why on earth would you put this on your poster for school?"

She simply replied, "Because I don't like it when you yell." I couldn't argue, it was me.

A few moms mentioned to me thereafter that they're "a yeller" too. I can't tell you it made me feel great to hear it, but I realized that my daughter was speaking her truth, and I needed to own mine. We all get fed up, and even when we try our hardest to make it work, sometimes things don't go as planned.

It's time we stop beating ourselves up for things like this, the honest truth of ourselves, but rather own our choices and learn from them. I've learned from this experience and I'm happy to say that I'm still not perfect. My kids know me well; I have days where I yell instead of speaking kindly all the time. I love the line my son gives me, accompanied by a big hug: "Mom, you're the best mom I ever had!" I chuckle and think to myself, "Thank goodness I'm the only one you've ever had or you might think differently."

Celebrate all of you, the good and the not-so-good, because in the end it's what makes you beautifully, uniquely YOU!

CHAPTER 3

Building Loving Relationships

I've been blessed many times over; I married my husband on September 23, 2000 and was absolutely delighted when our daughter joined the family in September 2002. I thought I knew the enormity of love the day I married my husband. Holding my daughter for the first time made me realize that love is limitless. I think every parent understands this the day they meet their new child. Our strong little boy followed along four years later and completed our family in November 2006. There is no greater blessing to be had in my life than these three people.

While the arrival of our son should have been one of the most joyous times in my life, it ended up being quite the opposite. Shortly after his arrival my body started expressing weird symptoms. I had made a pact with my sister-in-law to get in shape for our summer vacation together. We called it our "Summer-Sisters Bikini Pact": we'd get in shape and have to sport a bikini for one day of our beach vacation. I was motivated and ready to meet the challenge!

I'd hit the gym for an aerobic, cycling, or strength class and after returning home I'd end up in pain. First it was my elbow, then the shoulder, followed by knee or hip pain the next class. I've been a competitive athlete most of my life and although I knew something was "off" I really desired to push through the pain and get my body back into shape.

Before long, I found myself heading off to the rheumatologist; the pain I was experiencing wouldn't go away and in a short period of time it started to affect my well-being and overall functioning. I naively thought it'd be a quick and easy fix.

Months passed. By Christmas of 2007 I could no longer hold a pen or pencil, open a jar, or carry my son up the stairs. Simple, everyday tasks turned into acts of bravery. I would work through the pain while I washed my hair, pulled a shirt over my head, and brushed my teeth. The doctor ran a battery of tests but I never quite met all the criteria for a diagnosis. I was stuck in limbo.

Chronic pain impacts every area of your life. I no longer had patience with my husband or kids, small movements would bring tears to my eyes, and getting down on the floor to play was impossible most days. I was just getting by. On the worst days I would wake in the morning and cry. I would hope for a refreshing start, a pain-free waking experience after rest, but it didn't happen. On these days, Rob would give me a hug and lift my torso from the bed. I would sit in my pain and brace myself for the moment my feet hit the carpeted floor.

It's hard to realize the impact that this has on the loved ones around you when you're in the thick of things yourself. My husband would fall asleep next to a crying wife, and wake up to the same. The kids got the best of me that I could give at the time, but I knew that my best wasn't good enough for my own standards. I was riddled with guilt and fear that this would never get better.

Eventually chronic fatigue, constant stomach aches, brain fog, memory loss, headaches, and muscle weakness followed the joint pain. I continued to see doctors and travel to specialists in search of an answer. My son's first birthday came and went while my body continued to reach new heights of deterioration.

Through this time of trial, I didn't offer my body much love or grace. I was angry that it would do this to me, wishing for it to function differently. Some days I found myself literally screaming with frustration. It's been almost nine years now, and while I've learned a lot about relationships along the way, I've realized the relationship that needed the most care and attention was the one I have with my own body.

Loving Relationships

We often think of relationships as the connections we have with people in our life, but what about other relationships? Let's explore our personal relationships with food in general, and also the relationship we have with ourselves. I would argue that these two relationships are the foundation of a healthy relationship with everything and everyone else in life.

Answer the following questions as best you can by circling the first answer that comes to you. No need to ponder or analyze, just answer and go to the next question:

❋ ❋ EXERCISE: *Healthy Relationship Check List*

My relationship with food:

1. I love "white foods" (bagels, bread, pasta, crackers, cereal). YES   NO

2. I enjoy soda, sport drinks, or sugar in my coffee every day. YES   NO

3. I reach for food to comfort me. YES   NO

4. I experience cravings for sweet or salty foods. YES   NO

5. I eat my meals in quick fashion.	YES	NO
6. I tend to eat on the run.	YES	NO
7. I love to snack when I'm watching TV.	YES	NO
8. I wake up thinking about food.	YES	NO
9. I count calories.	YES	NO
10. I use the words "good" and "bad" about food, for example: "I ate really well all week and then was bad when we went away for the weekend."	YES	NO

My relationship with myself:

1. I am critical of my appearance.	YES	NO
2. I often use the words "life is crazy" or "I have no time."	YES	NO
3. I worry about what others think of me (my appearance, my actions, my opinions).	YES	NO
4. I rarely take time for myself.	YES	NO
5. I wish I was thinner.	YES	NO
6. I wish I looked younger.	YES	NO
7. I compare myself to others.	YES	NO
8. The number on the scale can make or break my day.	YES	NO
9. I have tried many different diets.	YES	NO
10. I am afraid of failing.	YES	NO

Now that you've circled your answers, tally all your "Yes" answers for each category and write your tally into each line, then add your tallies and fill in the total number:

My relationship with food: *"Yes" tally:_____*

My relationship with myself: *"Yes" tally:_____*

TOTAL:_____

The reason I have you tally your scores in each area, and then find your total altogether, is because I want you to connect with how often you stated yes to each of these questions, and overall. You see, even one "yes" answer indicates that you have room for more health and happiness in that relationship, and as your number of yeses goes up, the bigger the opportunity you have for growth.

My goal is for you to realize that it is possible to have a loving, supportive relationship with food and yourself. I know too well what a strained relationship can look like in each of these areas. There were more days than not when I hated my body, for its appearance, for its inability to perform, for it failing me. Instead of rejoicing about all that it provided me, I would criticize and expect more. And as far as the food relationship, well that was full of love and hate for most of my years. I constantly rebelled, doused myself in sugar and processed foods, depended on it to carry me through my stressful days, and expected nothing but greatness from my mind and body. These were huge expectations, and when my body wasn't doing the job, I got angry. Looking back, it seems downright ridiculous that I would function from this place; but I did. And I find that at some point in life, most people do.

Today, you have the opportunity to provide love, grace and care to each of these relationships. As you continue to venture through the book, I'll provide guidance on how to do so. Step one is to absorb this information without judgment, without guilt; just be present with it. Decide how you'd like to build on each of these relationships and write down your thoughts about how you'd like to show up in each area.

✳ ✴ EXERCISE: *Relationships Journal*

What does your current relationship with food look like?

_____

_____

_____

_____

_____

_____

What type of relationship do you desire to have with food?

_____

_____

_____

_____

_____

_____

_____

What does your current relationship with your body look like?

_____

_____

_____

_____

_____

_____

_____

What type of relationship do you desire to have with your body?

Hopefully as you've worked through this chapter and the exercises, you've come to realize that all areas of life affect our health.

Looking and feeling good is not just about dieting, or a specific relationship with food. While nutrition is a key factor to long-term health (we'll discuss this in depth in Section II), there's much more to consider. We're flipping dieting on its head to focus on what's most important for long-term health: nourishing your body in every aspect of life. No crash diets, no yo-yoing up and down, just simple daily changes that your body will love so much your choices will soon become a new lifestyle.

CHAPTER 4

Own Your Health

Doctors, I believe, have the best intention when treating the patient. Unfortunately I encountered too many who rushed to treat my symptoms with harsh drugs. When doctors didn't have a reason or answer for my failing body, they would tell me it was "all in my head" and that I was "just depressed." I would be handed a script for one medicine or another and be sent on my merry way. I knew this wasn't in my head, and while I might have been experiencing sadness and fear, depression was not the cause of my failing body.

There were multiple problems. In the first 16 months of my illness I was diagnosed with rheumatoid arthritis, palindromic rheumatism, and psoriatic arthritis. The main course of therapy suggested by doctors was for me to take methotrexate for the rest of my life. They shared the list of side effects with me and told me if it didn't work we would move on to something stronger. The doctors would say I needed to suppress my immune system so it would stop overreacting and attacking my joints. I walked away every time, knowing in my gut this wasn't the right path for me. The muscle weakness, brain fog, constant stomach aches and chronic fatigue, I was told, were unrelated to the autoimmune problems I was having.

We must all actively participate in our health, and make choices that serve us well. My health journey has helped me gain clarity about my participation, and consider how my choices either impacted me positively, or, in many cases, negatively. This chapter is going to help you explore your own participation in life, challenge you to think outside the box, and create healthy boundaries for yourself. It's time to stand in your power.

Take Ownership

"TAKING OWNERSHIP" is about acknowledging your state of health and recognizing that you have full claim, authority, and power to create a healthy body, mind, and life for yourself. It is yours for the taking and now is the time to make it happen.

I never once considered that I needed to take ownership of all aspects of my health until it deteriorated at such a fast pace that doctors told me to go home and prepare for "what was to come." They meant the slow progression of a disease that would take my life. News such as this takes your breath away. It caused my world to stop in its tracks, and made me take a deep look into what was happening.

At first, I blamed everything else for my ill state of health and questioned how I could be put through such hell. But after a couple months of my ranting, I started a big internal investigation and came to the conclusion that everything about my life was contributing to my fast deterioration. While I exercised pretty consistently, I had other things working against me. I always functioned at 100 miles per hour, putting everyone else's needs before my own, committing to things I didn't have time for, eating a lot of sugar and nutrient-void foods, drinking a few Diet Cokes a day to keep my energy up, staying up way too late and waking too early, worrying about what everyone thought of me versus living in my truth, and missing out on a lot of nutrient-rich veggies, beans, whole grains, greens, and nuts and seeds. I simply did not own my body, my mind, or my life. I existed and thought it'd all work out. I've learned that it doesn't happen. We must make daily effort to rise to the occasion, make intentional choices that serve us, and own every bit of our happiness, our health, and our life.

What part of your health do you need to take ownership of? Here's a little exercise to get your internal investigation off to a solid start. In this exercise, you identify your starting point, your barriers, what it means to you to get the job done, and the steps you'll take to make it happen.

⚛ EXERCISE: *Internal Investigation*

Answer the following questions as quickly as possible, no need to analyze:

1. *I always have good intentions but never really get around to*

    _____

2. *The three things that are holding me back from just getting it done are:*
    1. _____
    2. _____
    3. _____

3. *If I were to consistently accomplish my good intention, I would feel*

    _____

    _____

4. If I were to take my last breath today, I would regret not having done this for myself because

_____

_____

_____

5. If it is meant to be, its up to me! I will do these three things for the next 30 days to take ownership of this one area of my life:

    1. _____

    2. _____

    3. _____

The second part of the exercise is to share your details with one person who will provide positive encouragement to help keep you on track.

Lastly, keep your answers where you can read them daily; this is the best reminder to own your health and keep moving forward.

Intentional Choices

What if every choice you made came with ease and aligned with your needs in life? From as far back as I can remember, I couldn't make a decision to save my life. I remember dining out at restaurants as a young teen hardly able to decide on what I wanted to eat, worried about whether my dish would be as good as what anyone else ordered and if it wasn't I knew I might not enjoy dinner as much. In my twenties it was feeling anxious about decisions to meet friends, or stay in, or to break up a relationship or stay in it because I was too scared. I was wishy washy about everything, and wasted a great deal of my life in the process.

Looking back I realize that it wasn't the decision-making process per se that was the problem, it was the fact that I wasn't confident enough in myself to make a decision. Maybe I wasn't sure about what I truly wanted, even if it was deciding between the egg omelet or pancake breakfast. The other issue was that when I did make a decision, I would question it over and over again. I would worry about what someone thought, or if I offended anyone by not showing up for the event, and so on. There was no "ease" in this process.

I've realized through my journey that I have to understand what my priorities are, and intentionally make choices that honor my health and happiness. I encourage you to do the same, and to ask yourself the following question when it's time to make a decision:

"What does this provide me?"

⚛ EXERCISE: *What Does this Provide Me?*

This simple question can be used in all areas of life. You can extend this questioning to address key situations. Here are some examples of how you can gain clarity about whether your choice will feed you positively or negatively.

1. *Will this event/food/activity nourish me in some way, or cause me stress?*

2. *This activity/responsibility will take time; do I have the time to give at this point in my life?*

3. *Does this decision feed my health and happiness or negate it?*

4. *Does this decision move my business forward or just create busyness?*

Think about a situation or area of your life that you find challenging. Ask yourself "What does this provide me?" and expand on your thoughts with any of the questions above. Journal your findings here and explore whether the situation, person or event is feeding you in health and happiness, or possibly negating it.

Journal entry:

_____

_____

_____

_____

_____

_____

_____

_____

_____

_____

_____

_____

Making intentional choices is about honoring the needs of your body, your mind, and your spirit. I've had clients say, "Angie, that just seems selfish to only consider my needs when making decisions." Please understand that this isn't about being selfish, but rather getting a check on your selflessness and making sure the activities, people, and volunteering you commit to are going to align with your life priorities, health, and happiness. There may be times when a friend in need is going to trump the decision to honor your own life at that given moment, but these scenarios should be few and far between. The fact of the matter is that you cannot serve yourself, your family, or others in a healthy, loving way if you're depleted. Many of us extend ourselves far beyond our means, whether it's time, energy, money, emotional availability, or physical labor. This only carries you further away from the health and happiness you deserve.

Ask yourself the questions, get comfortable with the awkward-ness you might feel in doing so, and learn to honor your needs along the way. It's a beautiful gift to offer yourself and to the people you love and care about.

CHAPTER 5

Building Healthy Boundaries

J ust as there are foods that feed health or illness in the body, there are relationships, activities, habits, and life decisions we make that can either support us in health, or feed the progression of disease. It is necessary for us to build awareness in this area, identify how these areas of life serve us, and create healthy boundaries to honor our needs while prioritizing what's most important to us.

Healthy Boundaries

I can confidently say I didn't exercise many healthy boundaries until long after my diagnosis. The basic principles like wearing my seatbelt while driving and taking my contacts out before going to sleep were within my healthy boundaries, but there were plenty of other activities that fed illness in my body. I overpromised my time and energy, which were critical to me as the illness settled in. I'd say yes to everyone, volunteer for everything, and burn the midnight oil to make it all happen. And as a result I often felt tired, so I'd pop open a can of Diet Coke for a burst of energy. I was indeed a people pleaser, worrying about letting people down instead of living in my truth. All of these behaviors fed the illness in my body; this is why it's so important to create healthy boundaries.

If you've ever been to a Pilates class you'll understand the concept of working from the "core" outward. This is the same concept we'll follow when creating healthy boundaries. We're going to work in three layers: must-haves, negotiables, and infrequent/unnecessary. Our core is the foundation for creating the boundaries necessary to feed us health and happiness and consists of our must-haves: what is of greatest importance. This core circle may include family, pets, job, exercise, travel, and health.

Just outside of our core is the second layer. This second layer includes the negotiables in our life. Negotiables add value, but not without cost. Because they are negotiable, you could take them or leave them and they would not impact the overall joy you experience. This middle area may include social media or gaming, television, shopping, volunteering, etc. You'll need to assess whether these things are positively or negatively impacting your life.

The last layer to consider includes the people, activities, and events in your life that should be considered infrequent/unnecessary. Take inventory: what might not be serving you so well? Are there activities or traditions that you continue to move forward with that are negatively impacting your health or life? Are there people in your life who cause you undue stress or negativity? These are the things that must be given great consideration, and need to be scheduled less frequently or placed into the unnecessary category in order for you to manage stress and achieve optimal health.

We are each uniquely created and have our own way of dealing with stress and negativity, but none of us are untouchable. Stress and negativity greatly impact our lives unless we learn to manage them appropriately. One absolute in this process is to create necessary boundaries—and then we must follow through and honor our individual needs. Understand that what that may work well for one person can be like poison for another. There is a need for balance.

I had a client who served the Unites States of America through many deployments in a short window of time. She and I worked together after she was released from her duties due to medical leave. Cindy[1] is a vibrant, beautiful woman who loves to exercise and care for herself in a healthy manner. During one of our coaching sessions she disclosed that during exercise she'd often break down in tears and feel anxious. At the time, she participated in exercise that took place in a gym setting, but with the structure and competitive nature that often mirrored her military past. While exercise can be a healthy outlet for stress reduction, this was clearly not the case for her. Cindy worked to better balance her exercise routine to include calming exercise complimented by the structured exercise that often brought her to tears. Working in a couple days of yoga followed by a few days of her normal exercise routine proved to be the balance she needed. It allowed her to enjoy the structured, competitive environment without emotional releases taking place.

Keep in mind that the activity that helps one person reduce stress can have the opposite effect on another. You know yourself best; make choices that support you, your healthy boundaries, and goals.

EXERCISE: *Healthy Boundaries*

Fill in the Healthy Boundaries chart below. Consider all areas of your life: People, activities, relationships, career, exercise, food, and more. Let the list for each area continue to grow and expand as you increase your awareness and better understand how these things in life serve you.

1 All names have been changed to respect my clients' need for privacy.

Must Haves: These are the things in your life that are of greatest importance to you; your number one priority! This core circle may include things such as family, pets, job, exercise, travel, health, etc.

Negotiables: These seem to add some sort of value to you, but not without cost. This middle area may include things such as social media or gaming, television, shopping, or volunteering. You'll need to assess whether these things are positively or negatively impacting your life and plan accordingly.

Infrequent/Unnecessary: Are there activities or traditions that negatively impact your health or life? Are there people who cause you undue stress or negativity? These things must be given great consideration, and may need to be placed into the unnecessary category for you to manage stress and achieve optimal health.

Healthy Boundaries

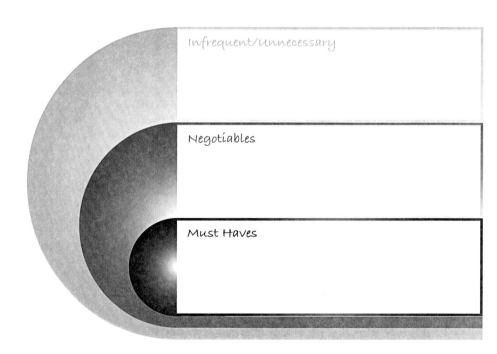

Infrequent/Unnecessary

Negotiables

Must Haves

Non-Negotiable

The word non-negotiable is direct, empowering, and leaves no room for error. It means there's no discussion to be had, no bargaining to take place, and no negotiation on the table. It provides instant communication about the topic or issue at hand, and allows everyone to move forward in quick fashion.

I've found this word to be useful in both my personal and professional life. When managing a team, they knew whether a topic was open for discussion, or not, by the use of this simple word. When grocery shopping with my kids, they know whether they can negotiate on a food item or not with the simple use of this word. It's immediately effective. I may have to provide the "why," but once they realize the food contains high fructose corn syrup, or a preservative that is non-negotiable, they understand and are empowered to make a healthier decision as well.

Another area of my life that has been served well by this word is my personal health. I have found that sometimes, in order for me to function from my healthiest place, I need to clearly identify the non-negotiables. The non-negotiables help me stay true to myself, my health, and my happiness.

Are there situations, people, activities, or expectations that feed unease or illness in your life? Through my journey, I realized it was necessary to close a relationship with a friend. I shared this with her, let her know that I cared for her and her family, and wished her many blessings for the future. But, I could no longer allow her negativity into my life. It was consuming me, and negating my health more than contributing to it. I didn't take this decision lightly, but I knew it was a non-negotiable in order for me to achieve health and happiness. Sometimes you have to do what's most difficult in order to move forward.

Other non-negotiables came up through my health journey. One was that we would not eat anything that contained high fructose corn syrup, as mentioned above. This specific ingredient feeds illness in the body, and had no place in our home. I'll never forget my daughter coming home from school one day, telling me that she didn't have the yogurt they were offered for a snack because it had high fructose corn syrup. She was in the third grade. My personal health rules and non-negotiables have carried over into the family, and as the years have passed, they've created a few of their own.

The non-negotiables, albeit few, come in handy. They provide a clear boundary and allow us to move forward. Take a few minutes to explore the situations, people, activities, or expectations that feed unease or illness in your life. Write them down here, and know that as you venture through this journey, you'll be filling your life and body with pure goodness. Often the activities and so on that negatively impact you will fall away while new, healthier habits take over. You'll recognize the need for non-negotiables as you go, and the few that do come up, you can honor by carrying out your new and improved healthy lifestyle.

✤ EXERCISE: *What Are My Non-Negotiables?*

My thoughts on the situations, people, activities, or expectations that feed unease or illness in my life:

_____

_____

_____

_____

_____

CHAPTER 6

Life Rules

In the summer of 2008 I was hospitalized for four days because I could not walk; not because I experienced paralysis, but because my leg muscles were struggling to hold me up. Leading up to the hospital stay I had experienced severe bouts of weakness accompanied by dizziness. After each episode I'd be thankful I had recovered.

One evening, though, I was standing at the stove making dinner when I felt the spell of weakness start. Before I knew it I was falling to the ground. I caught myself on the edge of the stove with my forearms and crawled along the countertop to the phone. I fell to the floor like a plop of Jell-O and phoned my husband. "Come home now," I told him. "Something is incredibly wrong." I army crawled over to my kids who were on the family room floor. With tears already streaming down my face and gripped with fear I lay near them and waited for my husband. We were off to the hospital in short order.

There were signs hung up all over the hospital room that said "High Risk Fall" and I was told not to get out of my bed without assistance. Doctors were in and out and tests were completed, including a two-hour full body CAT scan. I thought I could tough it out until they put the metal mask over my face. Into the machine I went. That's when I started to panic and hyperventilate; I continued pressing the help button as they rolled me out. They ended up giving me something to make me lie there without feeling anxious. While the tests weren't fun, I was getting used to being poked and prodded, all in the name of finding an answer. There had to be an answer.

While I lay in the hospital bed, I could often hear conversations between the nurses and doctors. Words like lupus, Multiple Sclerosis, Guillain-Barré, and more were tossed around. I was stumping doctors left and right. Although it was scary to hear the possibilities, in my heart I was hoping someone would find an answer. That had to be better than not knowing. I figured if an answer could be provided, so could a plan for a cure. I desperately wanted to have my old body back, be the energetic person I always was, and be the mom and wife I desired to be.

While I didn't have an answer at this time, I knew that my life was in need of change if I was going to get better. I was hardly functioning like I had in the past. In order for me to get well I would need to create healthy Life Rules to live by. These rules are positive and supportive, and have been my guide for many years now.

Creating Your "Life Rules"

Have you ever started something new, kept it going for a while, but eventually lost your "stick-to-itiveness"? Most people struggle with the ability to create life-long change and as a result, end up back in bad habits that negate health and happiness rather than nourish it.

In the previous chapter, you completed an exercise on healthy boundaries. Now I want you to create specific Life Rules. These Life Rules will be a positive, supportive foundation. They will serve as your guide to focus on the important things in life, honor the person you want to be, and allow you to function from your healthiest place.

Creating your personal life rules allows you to identify the things most important to you, and then follow up to nourish these priorities through your choices and actions. This document is your guide to achieving the life you deserve and desire! While some rule books (think sports, company policy handbook, and legal rules) may be tight and strict, your personal rule book should feel positive, supportive, and empowering.

✖ EXERCISE: *My Life Rules*

First, identify the areas of your life that need your time and attention in order for you to be healthy and happy. Examples may include: sleep, healthy eating, exercise, time with family, outings with friends, travel, etc.

These areas in my life need my time and attention in order for me to be healthy and happy:

_____

_____

_____

_____

_____

_____

_____

_____

Secondly, identify how you're honoring these priorities in your life today. Do you schedule time for these necessities or are they constantly dropping to the bottom of the list and lacking attention?

I honor these areas of my life by:

_____

_____

_____

_____

_____

_____

Next, ask yourself what it would provide you to give more time and attention to these areas of your life. Would you feel more rested and energized if you dedicated time for adequate sleep? Would you feel fulfilled because you were able to spend time with your family? Or maybe you would feel rejuvenated after a weekend camping in the woods. The choices we make either nourish us and provide stability in our life, or cause imbalance and hardship. Which category do your choices fall into?

By giving more time and attention to these areas of my life, I would be provided:

_____

_____

_____

_____

_____

_____

At times, we may do well balancing one area of our life, but lack in another.

List a minimum of four Life Rules that will guide you to the live the life you desire. Be specific and concise. For instance, if it's your goal to spend more time with friends because they showed up in your "core" of healthy boundaries, but in the life rules exercise you realize you're not doing as much as you'd like to foster these relationships, one of your Life Rules could be "I spend quality time with friends every month." Be as specific as possible; if you desire to be less judgmental then a life rule might be "I live a life without judgment and find grace in all circumstances." Create your Life Rules here and feel free to add as many as you'd like.

My Life Rules:

1. _____
2. _____
3. _____
4. _____
5. _____

Post your Life Rules where you'll see them every day; at your desk, on your mirror, or on the dash of your car. Create space in your calendar, if you're not already doing so, to carry out the necessary actions to honor your Life Rules. And finally, take time to celebrate your dedication and success.

You own your health and happiness! Take time to prioritize your needs, follow your Life Rules, and make choices that serve you.

CHAPTER 7

To Thy Self Be True

At the end of my four-day stay at the hospital, no answers were provided and I was sent home. I had a very difficult time with this roller coaster ride, so badly wanting someone to figure things out and provide direction. Time and time again I came up empty handed; sometimes I'd move on and stay positive while other times I'd crumble and fold. This was a time I crumbled.

You too may have a dark night of the soul; it's part of growing, releasing, and being able to move forward. Allow it to occur. Then take a quiet moment to decide how you'd like to respond in the future. Figure out the next step you're going to take in the process and go do it. Your feelings surely need to be acknowledged; and once they are please find the strength to move forward. You have it within you to do so.

My own break finally came in July of 2008.

I just wanted someone to listen, to care, and to have an open mind to do some research and find the answers I was so desperately looking for. I met my general practitioner at the point when muscle weakness already entered into the fold. He spent over an hour with me my first visit. He listened, he was interested, and at one point he pulled out the Physician's Desk Reference and started researching symptoms. He didn't have the answers, but I had new hope simply because he cared. He played a major role in my path to wellness because he provided a safe place; he advocated for me to get into a premier medical institution and in the end connected me with the man who would provide me a diagnosis.

This was a doctor who specialized in neuromuscular disease. I was anxious waiting in the patient room. He asked a lot of questions, listened to me share my story, and we explored my symptomology. And then he said something that changed me. It went something to the tune of: "Mrs. Gaffney, while I don't have the exact answers at this moment, I have some ideas of things we need to look into further. It'll take time and if you can be patient, we'll work as a team to figure all this out."

Calm came over me. I had finally found someone who had an idea of where to start! Best of all, he was in it for the long haul. He was ready to do the necessary work to figure out the problem, and he was asking me to be a part of his team! For the first time in a long time, I felt hopeful and ready to do whatever was necessary.

I thought back to all the other times I had left office after office without an answer. Sometimes my departure included the accusation that it was just all in my head, or that I needed to exercise to regain my health, or to take a medication to help the autoimmune symptoms. I knew in my heart of hearts, over and over again, that these were not the correct answers for me. There had to be someone who would listen and understand my needs. I knew my body better than anyone else on this planet. I stayed true to myself, even though it was difficult at times, and in the end I found what I was seeking.

Above All, to Thy Self be True

This seems like an easy one to check off the list. However, I find it one of the most challenging things to do. This concept requires a lot of attention, fact checking, and a strong commitment.

We all have a limiting belief system, meaning we think thoughts (true or not) that encourage us to respond in a certain way. Limiting belief systems can pull us away from our truth, and cause us to make decisions that don't serve us well at all. If you've ever had thoughts like, "I'm not good enough" or "I don't deserve this," or "How could he love me?" then you've experienced limiting self-talk which feeds our limiting belief system.

We all experience conditioning throughout our life. As a result of our interactions with mentors, parents, teachers, and even our own peers, we start to believe certain things about ourselves and create a response that suits the situation. Because of this conditioning and repeated response mechanism we develop limiting beliefs about ourselves and in turn do not always live in our truth.

It is not until we open ourselves to what we truly want that we will be able to attain it.

A client of mine suffered from Crohn's disease for many years before I met her. She experienced severe levels of chronic pain, had low energy, was often sad and impatient with life and was feeling desperate for change when we first met. Because of these symptoms and hardship over many years, she was conditioned to believe that she could no longer be healthy, and that she must accept this way of life for the rest of her days on earth. While it took months for her belief systems to change, I'm happy to announce that she's back to living life from the glass-half-full perspective, she smiles, she sees possibility, and she knows that her body is here to support her in this life. She's done amazing work to reduce inflammation, which in turn has allowed her to live with minimal to no pain. She's active again, going for walks in the evening, and enjoys fun on the Colorado River. She often tells me how people comment on how happy she looks.

The physical changes of weight loss, reduced pain and inflammation, better sleep, and clearer skin have all fed her ability to see the possibility, and open herself to a life of health and happiness. But it didn't come without a lot of emotional focus and support. There were plenty of days where the limiting beliefs and limiting self-talk would cause her to fumble or lose sight of her truth. People would question her about her new eating habits, or ask for her to help with activities that were still too demanding for her healing body. She learned to use her voice and live in her truth in order to make decisions that supported her healthy, vibrant life.

What's holding you back from living in your truth? Start journaling your thoughts around this question. Consider the conditioning you've had in your childhood or later in life that has held you back from living in your truth.

❊ EXERCISE: *My Truth*

What's holding you back from living in your truth?

What conditioning have you received throughout life? Were you trained to never speak up? Were you raised to question your value and worth? Our conditioning helped shape us into who we are today. Sometimes, the conditioning doesn't serve us well in adulthood even though it may have had a purpose in childhood. Please travel back in time, consider your childhood, the teenage years, when you were off to college and on your own and even young adulthood.

What challenges did you face and how did your conditioning feed these challenges?

_____

_____

_____

_____

_____

_____

_____

_____

What would it look and feel like if you could freely speak and live your truth? Where you have no worries about what others may think, or whether your truth might ruffle someone's feathers?

_____

_____

_____

_____

_____

_____

_____

What first step do you need to take to start living in your truth?

_____

_____

_____

_____

_____

Do the Thing You Shouldn't Do

Do you have a need to please? I sure as heck did for a lot of years, and let me tell you its hard trying to carry out the "perfect" life! It's also not healthy or realistic.

So many of us place expectations on ourselves to do the right thing and practice perfection. But how does this really serve us? How does this add calm and allow you to live in your truth? If you're like the old me, you probably answer every phone call that comes in, follow up on every text immediately, and answer emails a hundred times a day. You say yes to most, if not all, requests and give beyond your physical and emotional means.

We live in a place where instant communication, immediate gratification, and social media are the norm. But what would happen if we create our own "norm" and start taking control of our lives instead of having life control us?

Starting today, I want you to do one thing you believe you shouldn't do. This may include letting a call go to voicemail and tending to it later, it may mean having a bite of dark chocolate after lunch, or skipping the gym because your body is telling you it needs a day off.

My kids are old enough now where sports and extracurricular activities consume our evenings. While it's fun to see them active and involved, I experienced a bit of anxiety trying to get from one place to the next in a timely manner. Even when it wasn't physically possible, I got uptight about being late. This was not a favorable moment in our house; I would yell and get upset that we couldn't find the other soccer shoe, or the book we needed, or whatever the case might be. After a while, I realized that this wasn't serving anyone in a healthy manner. The kids would be upset, and I would feel angry and frustrated because the shoe wasn't in the bin as I instructed.

I had to finally let it go. No more yelling, no more anxiety, we do our best to get to our activities on time and if we're late...well, we're late. When we do our best and accept what is, life seems to run smoothly. I still try to make sure the soccer shoes are ready the night before, and the book is in the library bag ready to go, but in the event something sets us behind I say to my kids and myself, "We do our best always, and today our best means that we're going to be 10 minutes late." We strive to be on time, and I'd say 97% of the time we make our goal; the other 3% of the time we keep our cool and arrive when we arrive. We're all better for it, and the kids have mentioned over and over that they love their "calm mom." I believed for a very long time that someone would think poorly of me for arriving late, when in fact most people understand. The best part is that I feel confident enough in myself and my boundaries that if they don't understand, I'm okay with it. They have the right to feel whatever they want, but it's not my job to worry about it.

The same goes for you. Always do your best, knowing that your best may look different from one day to the next, and that is perfectly okay.

Do one thing you think you shouldn't this week! Let the call go to voicemail, stay in your pajamas all day, don't sweat the small stuff, and know that you're amazing just the way you are. In fact, you're already doing something you "shouldn't do," and that is ditching the diet and instead, cultivating amazing relationships in your life; with food, with your body and with others. Getting comfortable with yourself and your new lifestyle will mean letting go of the small stuff, not worrying about what you "should do" and going after what you know will serve you best.

Now go be a rebel and enjoy every minute of it!

CHAPTER 8

Be Vulnerable

In the months following the first visit with my specialist I completed a lot of tests. The doctor thought I most likely had mitochondrial disease or Lyme disease. Preliminary results seemed to point toward mitochondrial disease, and after a few months of waiting, the nurse called me to schedule a follow-up appointment. She told me the test results were all in and the doctor knew what was wrong. He could see me on November 4, 2008. This date is significant now for two reasons, but the main reason is that it is my son's birthday. I would finally get my answer on my son's second birthday!

A Different Perspective

The morning of November fourth was different than most. I found the energy to shower and get dressed in a nice outfit. I did my hair and even threw on a little make-up. I wanted to be feeling great for this day; I had waited to get an answer for far too long. Today I would begin healing. I felt so confident that I even told my husband he didn't need to come. I made the one-hour drive to the office and excitedly awaited my meeting with the doctor.

My doctor and the Physician Assistant came in to find me all smiles. He said, "We have some good news, and some bad news.

"The good news is that we know what is going on; you have mitochondrial myopathy. The bad news is that it is a progressive disease; it'll attack your various organs, cause droopy eye lids, diabetes, blindness, deafness and paralysis."

Somehow, I managed to keep it together. "Will this take my life?" I asked. He said that he didn't know of any good outcomes, and that I'd need to go home and prepare. He told me there was no way to predict how long the progression would take, but said that we caught the disease in its earlier stages and he was going to give me some supplements to help slow the progression.

The one-hour drive home was a difficult one. I could barely see the road in front of me, not because it was raining but because there was a storm of tears running from my eyes. Why me? What did I do to deserve this? How can I plan for what's to come? What do I tell my husband? How can I be a mom to my children while deteriorating to nothing? My mind was flooded with a lot of "what if's" and "why's" and "how's". Then I realized something about 15 minutes from home....a voice inside my head said, "Get yourself together, girl, you are headed home to celebrate your boy's birthday!" I put on my happy face, and we celebrated our sweet boy as he turned two.

The next morning, I did exactly as my doctor prescribed; I started researching mitochondrial myopathy. There was minimal information available at the time and most of what I read was people's blogs or articles about a person's journey with mitochondrial myopathy. Hearing about other failing bodies and death did me no good. I cried nonstop for days.

In my research I uncovered that children can be affected. After making a call, my doctor ran tests to see if I had the genetic mutation. It took a few weeks of waiting before it was confirmed that I did not. My kids were safe from the hereditary risk. What a blessing! But the question still existed, why and how on earth did I end up with this rare disease?

My doctor didn't know, so while we had the answer to what was going on, we didn't know why. My days were filled with thoughts of deterioration, and I started focusing on how to die gracefully. Before I would fall asleep at night I'd question whether I should write letters to my kids for their birthdays. I'd cry when I thought about missing out on the big events...my son going to kindergarten, my daughter heading to prom, being there the day they each got married and missing out on being a grandmother. Then thoughts would turn to my husband. How would he handle this all on his own? It was overwhelming; sadness, grief and fear filled my heart daily.

This news of needing to go home to prepare for a disease to progress and take my life completely consumed me. Not only did I think about the days I might not be here, and how I could share my voice with my family long after I was gone, I started thinking about how I'd lived my life up to that point. Did I savor enough moments, did I explore the places I wanted to explore, and did I say "I love you" enough?

If you were given this exact news today, how would you answer these same questions? Life gives us many opportunities to feel vulnerable, to rise to the occasion, and savor every beautiful moment.

Do Something that Scares the Tuna Salad Out of You!

We were in Kauai with a group of friends and we decided to go on a day trip of zip lining, swimming, and picnicking. We had guides showing us the way; we started small (or short in the case of the zip lines) and met the challenge of longer, higher lines as the day went on. I remember feeling nauseated a bit when stepping up to do the first zip line, and then quickly realized that my irrational fear was squelched by a quick ride that I found enjoyable. I was excited to see what else was to come.

While I greeted all future zip lines with determination, my anxiety got the best of me when we stopped for lunch and a swim. You see, I can handle a nice clean pool where you can see to the bottom, know how deep the water is, and can swim to the edge to hop out in easy fashion. This pool, however, was anything but my inviting description. It was a natural water hole; the water looked black and the only way to get in was to hike up the side of a cliff with the rest of my friends and jump off.

I followed my husband and group of friends up the small cliff; I was second-to-last. My stomach was a mess, my head full of fear, and my legs were weak. This was not my idea of fun. Everyone else jumped, and after stepping up for my turn, I froze. Our friend Scott was behind me, cheering me on with his never-ending positive smile. All the friends already in the water were hooting and hollering for me to hop on in, telling me that it'd be okay. But the fear, that damn fear, filled my body. I felt my heart racing, my breath shallow, and thought of the creatures that might be living in the black water. I think I've watched too many shows on water snakes and other lovely creatures with my animal-loving children. This education wasn't coming in handy!

Scott asked me if he should give me a push, which I quickly responded no to. I knew I had to jump on my own. After many minutes, which felt like an eternity to me, I jumped…and guess what? I survived! I actually did it! I raced to my inner tube, and once I was securely on top of it, I made sure my toes stayed out of the water (because of course if there were snakes, they'd bite my toes). I can't say I relaxed for any amount of time, but I stayed. I tried to enjoy the time with my husband and friends, and got out when it was time to enjoy lunch.

What may seem an easy, fun experience to some is the fear of death to another. It's funny how we're all wired differently. Not one other person in our group struggled with this jump into the dark water, just me. I was slightly embarrassed, but more than that I was incredibly proud of my choice to step through the fear and do it. It provided me the opportunity to experience something I'll probably never have the chance to do again. It allowed me to take part in the group activity and share in the fun memory. And in the end, I would've been much more regretful that I missed out, versus stepping through the fear and getting the job done.

I'd like to thank all the water snakes for leaving me alone that day, and all my friends and husband for the support they provided. That moment will be a cherished memory for the long haul.

My challenge to you today is to also do something that scares the tuna salad right out of you. You may feel sick, weak in the knees, and ready to crap your pants, but in the end you'll feel like you can handle anything that comes your way...even the greatest of fears!

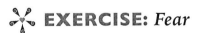 EXERCISE: *Fear*

Can you think of a time or experience when fear set in and caused you to change your course of action?

Write about that experience, how you felt, and how your decision was based on fear:

_____

_____

_____

_____

_____

What did you miss out on, how did you feel after allowing the fear to determine your fate, and did you realize after the fact that your fear was irrational?

_____

_____

_____

_____

_____

_____

What would you like to do in the next few months to overcome a great fear? Maybe it's singing in the church choir, talking to your boss about a work situation, or running your first 5K race... whatever it is for you, I want you to think big, and write out a plan to take action. You may feel sick to your stomach and weak in the knees when it comes time to execute; just remember that you will overcome. Even if the worst-case scenario happens, you'll feel accomplished and free as a result of conquering a fear that has held you back in one way or another.

Write your plan here: What will you do to overcome a fear in the coming months? Identify the fear you'll overcome, and write out your plan to do so.

_____

When the day comes, try belly breathing (more about breathing in Chapter 24), and recite positive words of encouragement to yourself with the in-breath and release the negative thoughts and fear on the outbreath. Fear can exist anywhere; you may even feel vulnerable about the changes you want to make for your health. This is a natural response, and you can use these same tools when you experience this. Always remember your end goal, and start with that in mind as you work through changes to nourish your body at the table and in life. You've got this. I'm so proud of you for rising to the occasion and fulfilling this activity for yourself.

CHAPTER 9

Nourishment for the Soul

Whatever we plant in our subconscious mind and nourish with repetition and emotion will one day become a reality. ~ Earl Nightingale

A perspective can change depending on the lens through which you see it. The color of my lens changed often throughout my health journey. Some days it was dark gray, cloudy and thick, and on a rare occasion I found myself looking through a pretty clear lens. And there were plenty of days where I wore every shade in between. As you can imagine, I had a very difficult time seeing anything beyond the lens when it was dark gray and cloudy. I couldn't see the bright light or beautiful colors that surrounded me, but instead was singularly focused on all the negativity and challenge in my life.

It's amazing to me how much your life can change when there's a shift in perspective. Through the years of healing, and gaining a better understanding of my body, I've been able to express more gratitude, focus on the positive in any situation and quickly know when it's time to take off the dark gray lens and replace it with the clear one. What lens do you find yourself wearing most often? Do you tend to see things in a negative or challenging way, or are you able to find celebration, gratitude and grace in all situations?

A Place of Gratitude

There is no greater place to live than in a place of gratitude.

The simple practice of giving thanks can create a life-changing shift in perspective and happiness. I was lucky enough to be taught about gratitude in my childhood years, but honestly never truly practiced it on a consistent basis until two years ago. This is when I started to realize that practicing gratitude creates a larger shift than just having a grateful heart.

How many times in your life have you stewed over a situation, or fed emotions with negative fuel that held you in a place of sadness, anger, or doubt? It's almost too easy to get caught up in this pattern, but each of us has the ability to choose differently, and feed the mind with good. When we're able to do this consistently, life gets brighter, happier, more calm and balanced.

One of the most beautiful gifts of living in a place of gratitude is the awareness you build for all the small happenings in life. You'll begin to notice more beauty in nature, in people, in your relationships, and even in times of hardship. You capture the yummy smells, home cooked meals, sweaty sons and daughters who've been out to play all day, and the scent of your partner's skin as you embrace one another. These are some of the small happenings that often get left behind in the fast-paced world we live in. Living in a place of gratitude allows you to stop, build awareness, and celebrate all the beauty in your life.

Begin your own daily practice of gratitude and note how shifts in your life begin to take shape.

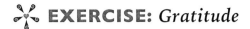

EXERCISE: *Gratitude*

Select a journal to be used only for your gratitude practice.

Every night before bed write out a list of 10 things you're grateful for. These can be "things" both big and small.

When you wake each morning, take a brief moment to give thanks. You can give thanks for anything your heart desires.

Last but not least, while looking in the mirror each morning take a moment to give thanks and gratitude to your amazing body.

Write daily or weekly notes in your journal about changes that occur in your life as a result of this practice.

Inspire Others and Share Your Gifts

Each of you has amazing gifts to share with this world, and it's time to share them! I want you to think about experiences, situations, activities, and skills that seem to come easy to you, or that you've learned from and you have passion for. Maybe it's singing, working with children, organizing people's homes, creating websites, or helping fundraise for nonprofit organizations. Your gifts are both large and small, and often we don't even see them as a gift we have to offer, but rather something that just comes easily to us. When we have the opportunity to share our passion and gifts with others we experience great joy and fulfillment in our own lives, just as the recipient does.

What are your gifts? This can be a challenging question for some, but believe me, the gifts are there! Take a few minutes, and declare your gifts below.

Don't be shy about this exercise. It's time you celebrate the gifts you've been given and use them to inspire others. I never thought of my health journey as a gift until I was well out of the dark hole of illness and on the road to healthy, vibrant living. I hardly saw past my own nose in the difficult days, but once the healing process started I began to realize that this was a gift I'd been given, to hold and treasure and in the end share with others.

Not everyone has to go through a life journey to identify their gifts. Identify what you're passionate about and who you'd like to share your gifts with. Maybe it's an expertise you can put to work and share through a career, or maybe it's something that will serve a volunteer organization perfectly. There are endless opportunities. The starting point is identifying your gifts, so do it right now. List three.

Step two: Celebrate these gifts, have the courage to step out in a way that may take you out of your comfort zone, and share them. It'll be one of the most fulfilling things you do.

✂ EXERCISE: *My Gifts*

Three gifts I'd like to focus on are:

1._____
2._____
3._____

The gift I will focus on first is _____
and I'd like to share it by:

_____

_____

_____

_____

_____

As an example, maybe the gift you'd like to focus on first is singing and your goal is to share your singing with others. You know of a group that sings Christmas carols for various nursing home audiences and this is how you decide you'll inspire others through your gift of singing. Take the appropriate steps to engage the singing group and get involved.

If you experience any fear around this task, take a step back and refer to the breathing technique in Chapter 24. On each in-breath recite to yourself: "I am enough," "I know enough," and "I'm here to share my gifts." On each exhale, allow all the negative thoughts and fear to release from you. You're ready to do this; you have everything you need and you're ready to spread love, joy, and your talents with the world to enhance the lives of others. There's no greater gift than this.

I believe with every part of my being that you'll rise to the occasion and in the end feel empowered and filled with incredible joy! Feel free to correct me if I'm wrong.

This concludes Section I! Now that you've worked on giving your #1 fan the love and care it needs to support you, it's time we move on to building a solid foundation. You'll hear me say it time and time again; the foundation of health begins with food. But not just any food. In the following chapters, I'll cover nutrition basics, dive into the importance of food, and how to select the best fare to keep you healthy for life. There's a method to the madness, and it's important to me that you always understand the "why" behind the strategies and principles I suggest. Stick with me through the details, knowing that it'll serve you well. You'll also find many resources in the back of the book to assist you in further research.

SECTION II

Building a Solid Foundation

Building a solid foundation largely involves the food you eat to nourish the body. In the beginning of the book I shared that we would focus on both table food and life food to help you achieve optimal health. This section of the book is focused on table food. Honestly, if there was only one thing I could choose to do for the rest of my life to ensure my best chances of living a healthy, high quality life it would be to eat whole, nourishing foods to support my body. I know all too well that if my cells aren't happy, my organs aren't either, and eventually it leads to illness. So let's gear up to build a solid foundation for long-term health.

You're going to explore a lot of information and be challenged to assess your current habits with food. Take time to get through this section. Reflect on the exercises and be open to new ideas. These pages will provide you practical tips and tools you can implement to create ease in your life. Above all else, be kind to yourself through the process. We all do what we know and when we know more, we can do even better. It's how life goes. Even after almost seven years of being on my health journey, I'm still learning and doing better each and every day to build the solid foundation. Give yourself permission to do the same.

CHAPTER **10**

It Starts with Food

The foundation of health begins with food; it's as simple as that. If only I knew it was that simple before I got ill.

I honestly don't know if I would've listened even if someone had told me; my husband begged me to get the sugar out of the house and that didn't work. It was at the deepest point of desperation that I began to research food and tried to learn how it could help me. I learned facts about what an antioxidant does, which foods harm your cells, and how the right food can truly help your body heal.

The next step was putting some of my reading into action. I changed my eating and started slowly feeling the benefit of doing so. I took all these teachings into my studies as a Certified Health Coach. My holistic team also shared their thoughts as my journey continued. I had support from every angle telling me the truth about food. On the one hand it seems so simple, and yet on the other it doesn't because we're trained to think differently.

Medicine is necessary at times, but it's not the end-all, be-all answer, and most often it doesn't address the root cause of the health issue. The body thrives on whole food nourishment. Your cells get what they need to function at their best, and your organs too! The key to success is filling up on phytonutrient-rich plant foods that fight disease in the body, boost your immune system, and keep you looking young and vibrant. I do understand how this can be a challenge in our fast-paced world and we'll be addressing this in the following chapters too.

One of the best comments I received from a client had to do with this fact, that food is the foundation of health. He carried excess weight, had a horrible time sleeping, often experienced moodiness, and lacked energy every day. About two months into the coaching, he said, "Angela, I can hardly believe that I've lost weight, I'm sleeping through the night, and I feel so energetic!" He went on to say that if I had told him that he would've experienced all this just by changing how he ate, and hydrating well, he never would've believed it. The best thing is that he never felt deprived, or restricted, but rather empowered through the work he did. I hope the same for you!

Not Always Easy

Throughout my journey, I've made a lot of changes. It began with changing the way I ate; clearing out all the harmful processed foods and replacing with organic whole foods. Thereafter, I learned to start saying no, removed toxic house cleaners from my home, replaced all my nonstick cookware and more.

These changes all took place over time, working on one area before moving on to the next. While my husband was incredibly supportive and encouraging me every step of the way, there were people in my life who didn't quite understand or welcome all the change. Being healthy isn't always an easy task. People would question why I was doing something. They would disagree with my need to rid my body of the foods that were hurting it, and seemed impatient at times.

One thing that has happened over time is that I rarely enjoy alcohol anymore. I might have a small glass of wine at an event, but the days of just having a glass in the evening are far gone. I'm not suggesting that you need to do this; it's just something that I've needed to do for myself. I've been amazed how much time and effort people have invested in trying to sell me on the need to drink; at times I've felt like I was back in junior high getting peer pressured into doing something I didn't want to do.

I had to come to terms with the fact that this was my way of life; the life I've chosen to create for myself and my family. I need not explain to anyone why I choose not to drink, or maybe why I have chosen to do so if I do indulge in a glass of wine. People may feel uncomfortable at times because of my choices. I share this with you because you may encounter something similar in your own journey.

We can't control how others respond; but we can hold true to what we know is good and right for us and decide how we want to participate in life, no matter the situation. You've gone through the healthy boundary exercise, and have created your Life Rules to serve as your guide. I'd like you to take a few minutes to explore your new way of life. Has everyone supported you along the way? Have you felt resistance, or experienced any challenges? Please share your thoughts here.

EXERCISE: *My New Life*

_____

_____

_____

_____

_____

_____

_____

_____

_____

_____

_____

_____

_____

Each of us has the power to create the life we want to live; to honor the needs of our body, mind and spirit, and to do it all without the need for explanation. It is my wish that you get cozy with your way of life, celebrate all that it brings you, and feel confident in every choice you make. Allow others the permission to respond however they need to respond, and move forward knowing that you're creating the life you desire.

In the next chapter we'll dive into specific dietary information, including information on various nutrients. This is where you'll learn the secret to flipping dieting on its head! I know I get a little sciency (is that even a word?) with you in the following chapters; stick with it and you'll have a great understanding of why food is the foundation of health.

CHAPTER **11**

Food as Fuel

The diagnosis proved to be a big struggle. I'd spend hours every day researching mitochondrial myopathy, trying to understand what it meant for me. In my research I'd come across chat rooms for people with various neuromuscular diseases and I remember talking to my husband about joining an online group of people who suffered from mitochondrial myopathy. He very matter-of-factly said, "Why would you spend your time with people who also have failing bodies instead of focusing on something that'd bring you joy?" I think that was the beginning of my light bulb moment. I woke up one day and literally said to myself, "To hell with figuring out how to die gracefully, I'm going to learn how to live!"

I switched gears with my hours of research, and started finding information on foods that could help my cells. I had heard about antioxidants before, but had no clue what they actually did. I researched everything under the sun about preservatives, toxins, artificial sweeteners, sugar, and more, and realized something big. Really BIG. In all my life, I had never considered the quality of my food, but rather was always focused on the quantity. I had counted calories, restricted calories, went without carbs, with carbs, high protein, low fat, no fat and more. I had participated in weight loss programs, read plenty of diet books and would yoyo up and down all the time.

This health journey has been a treasured gift for many reasons; having a new relationship with food is one of the many gifts I've been given. In this chapter, you'll learn the basics of food, why it's so important to consider the quality over quantity, and assess whether all calories are equal.

The Daily Essentials

Many people come to me already on a diet, are afraid of fat, think they need to be eating only low calorie foods, or skip carbohydrates and beef up on protein. We are all different and have unique needs when it comes to nourishing our body. However, there are some very basic principles that should guide us.

Most people have a restrictive, guilt-ridden, love-hate relationship with food. We've dieted, and been "good" with our eating and then fallen off track and eaten poorly; yo-yoing up and down all the while. There are over 1,000 new diet books that hit the shelves every year; most of these focus on restricting one of the three macronutrients. There's the low carb diet, the high protein diet, the no fat diet, the zone diet and others. Diets are built on restriction, deprivation, guilt, and plenty of other negative emotions. **This book is not a diet book**; we're going to build a healthier relationship with food and your body.

The healthiest way to nourish our bodies is to eat a diet balanced with macronutrients, robust in micronutrients, and overflowing with phytonutrients. If I ask a crowd of people, "What is the most important factor of any diet?" there is one consistent and overwhelming answer I receive, and that is…drum roll please…calories. CAL-OR-IES! We hear about them everywhere we turn, but should they be the main focus of our diet? Let's first explore a few nutrients and then return to this important question.

The three types of nutrients we'll cover are Macronutrients, Micronutrients, and Phytonutrients. I know this isn't the most exciting text in the book, but stick with me because understanding these three types of nutrients will be key to your long-term success.

The strategies I share with you are not a "diet," but rather a way of life that doesn't require guilt, restriction, deprivation, or will power. You'll fuel the body with energy, support healing, proactively fight disease, and transform your life.

Macronutrients include protein, fat and carbohydrates; the three primary food groups that we get energy from. Macronutrient consumption is essential for living, and if omitted from the diet, the body will experience adverse effects. I want you to consider the comments I made earlier about dieting; people tend to focus on this category of food when they are on a diet. There are even diets that focus on balancing these food groups. I've done plenty of them, and felt restricted and deprived and in the end fell right back into my old habits.

Have you also dipped into dieting? How did the diet focus on protein, carbohydrates, and fat? Finding a diet book that will work well for you is like finding a needle in the haystack.

Micronutrients include vitamins and minerals; each is necessary for longevity and quality of life, but we need them in "micro" or small amounts; our body depends on these for physiological functions. Micronutrients are abundant in whole foods, and as food is processed these micronutrients can be compromised or void. It is essential to include micronutrient-rich foods in your daily diet to support the functioning of your body. Everyone plans to live for a long time; your micronutrient-rich foods will provide you a good quality of life so you're able to enjoy all your days as you continue to age.

Before reading on I want you to "put up your dukes"—that's right, make two fists and hold them up like you're ready to fight. C'mon, nobody is watching... do it! This is the image I want in your mind when you think about our next group of nutrients, phytonutrients (pronounced Fight-o-nutrients). What a cool name for this group of nutrients! Here's why it's the coolest name: because this group of nutrients is like having the largest military force inside your body to fight off all the enemies that cause disease. And as a bonus, when you eat the foods that contain these powerful phytonutrients, you'll not only feed health into your body, but you'll lose weight, have more energy and feel amazing. Now these are the kind of side effects any of us would gladly welcome into life. Here's the scoop on your military force:

Phytonutrients can also be called phytochemicals. These are chemical compounds that naturally occur in plants and are responsible for the color, taste, and smell of foods. For instance, phytochemicals are responsible for the deep purple color of blackberries, which also provides the body antioxidant benefits. Although phytochemicals have not been established as an essential nutrient by the US FDA, they are known to offer antioxidant immune-boosting and disease-prevention benefits to the body. Phytonutrients are abundant in plant-based foods (think of anything that comes from our earth: leafy greens, vegetables, fruit, whole grains, beans, nuts, seeds). The more color you add to your plate, the more opportunity you have to consume these wonderful chemical compounds and enrich your life. Be creative with your food and think about the rainbow when making your food choices: purple, blue, red, orange, yellow, green, and you can add in pink, peach, and brown too!

As I mentioned earlier, most traditional diets focus on the macronutrient category. They tend to increase, lower, or sometimes omit one of the classes of food in order to achieve a weight-loss benefit. I too have previously taken part in the low-carb diet, the low-fat and no-fat diet, and high protein diet. While you may receive a short-term boost from the change in daily diet, these options are not sustainable for life nor do they provide you the balance your body needs. It's time we turn things upside-down with dieting and focus instead on the phytonutrient category to lead the way. The fact of the matter is that if your diet is rich in phytonutrient foods you'll be getting all the disease-fighting properties you need, and by default you'll receive most of the micronutrients you need and still be able to balance your macronutrient intake. Easy, effective, and a perfect plan to achieve health and longevity. That's it folks. We flip dieting on its head by moving macronutrients to the bottom of the priority list and phytonutrients to the top. When you do so, you'll automatically feel much better, and achieve your health goals.

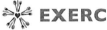 EXERCISE: *My Food*

In this exercise, I need you to be honest and truthful with yourself. Throughout this book, you'll have a lot of opportunity for self-reflection and growth, which can lead to some negative thoughts and self-judgement. When any negative thoughts or feelings come up as a result of the exercises in this book, please remind yourself that you're not here to judge, or be demeaning to yourself in any way, but rather to honor the fact that there may be opportunity to grow, and create more health and happiness in your life. The only way we can do this, is to explore what is working and that which might not be working so well.

Please answer the following questions by selecting "Yes" or "No":

1. I eat 3 meals a day.	YES	NO
2. I eat 2 cups of fruit daily.	YES	NO
3. I eat at least 4 cups of vegetables daily.	YES	NO
4. In addition to my vegetables, I eat 2 cups of leafy greens daily.	YES	NO
5. I eat an ounce of nuts or seeds daily.	YES	NO
6. I eat whole grains daily.	YES	NO
7. I enjoy green tea daily.	YES	NO
8. I consume ½ cup of beans 5 days a week.	YES	NO
9. I eat salmon at least once a week	YES	NO
10. I regularly use olive oil and/or coconut oil.	YES	NO
11. I rarely eat fast food.	YES	NO
12. I cook from scratch.	YES	NO
13. I do not crave sweets.	YES	NO
14. I drink 64+ oz of water daily.	YES	NO
15. I drink less than two cups of coffee per day.	YES	NO
16. I have never been on a diet.	YES	NO
17. I do not count calories.	YES	NO

If you've answered "no" to any of the statements in this exercise, you have the opportunity improve your health and happiness through diet alone. As you continue through the book, you'll receive strategies to support you incorporating more phytonutrient-rich foods into your diet and let me tell you, you're going to LOVE how you feel as a result! Nice work with this exercise. Give yourself some love now and express gratitude for your honesty, your big heart and your desire to do your best in health and happiness.

CHAPTER 12

Macronutrients

Let's dive a bit more into the three macronutrients before our calorie discussion. This brief overview should help you understand how carbohydrates, protein, and fat each serve the body in health. It is very important to balance these three categories of food for optimal health, but it's just as important to make sure we're selecting the highest quality macronutrients as well.

Carbohydrates, protein, and fat make up the group of macronutrients. These are the food groups that often take center stage with traditional diets. However, each plays a critical role in health and if you omit any one food group there's going to be a breakdown in the functioning of your body.

People often focus on these food groups in misleading ways; me included. I think I practiced the low-fat diet for a couple of years and I loved it! I got to eat all the foods I was addicted to: low-fat Snackwell cookies, no-fat ice cream, bagels, pasta, and Diet Coke! I followed the diet pretty easily and stayed thin. However the long-term consequences would far outweigh any benefit it ever provided me. Beyond feeding my sugar addiction, it also fed inflammation in my body. I didn't have enough fat to absorb fat-soluble vitamins, and was void of many micronutrients. Not to mention barely consuming phytonutrients. I didn't even know the word phytonutrient existed back then. This is the reason I wanted to shed new light on that amazing group of food. We need each one to create a healthy body; but you do need to be selective about the types of food you consume in each category, so that's where we'll start.

Carbohydrates

The primary function of carbohydrates is to provide energy for the body, especially the brain and the nervous system. An enzyme called amylase helps break down carbohydrates into glucose (blood sugar), which is used for energy by the body. Carbohydrates include sugar, starches, and fiber.

Carbohydrates are classified into one of two categories: simple or complex. The classification depends on the chemical structure of the food, and how quickly the sugar is digested and absorbed. Simple carbohydrates have one (single) or two (double) sugars. Complex carbohydrates have three or more sugars.

Simple Carbohydrates: Single and Double Sugars

Single sugars include:

- Fructose (found in fruits)
- Galactose (found in milk products)

Double sugars include:

- Lactose (found in dairy)
- Maltose (found in certain vegetables and in beer)
- Sucrose (table sugar)

Honey is also a double sugar. But unlike table sugar, it contains a small amount of vitamins and minerals. (Note: Honey should not be given to children younger than 1 year old.)

Table sugar, candies, cakes, and cookies all fall into the "Simple Carbohydrate" category. These foods must be eaten in moderation because they lack the vitamins, minerals, and nutrients needed to nourish the body.

Eat lots of fruits and vegetables as simple sugars for good energy. They naturally provide your body the nutrients needed for healthy living.

Complex Carbohydrates: Three or More Sugars (often referred to as "starchy" foods)

- Dark leafy greens (kale, romaine, Swiss chard, spinach)
- Legumes
- Starchy vegetables
- Whole grains (brown rice, quinoa, oats)
- Whole-grain breads and cereals

Complex carbohydrates contain high amounts of fiber and take longer to digest than simple carbohydrates. They are also full of vitamins, minerals and nutrients to provide the body great energy, keep you feeling satiated, and fight disease.

"Good Carbs Versus Bad Carbs" Dilemma

Focus on carbohydrates that are whole foods; whole grains, vegetables, fruit, leafy greens, and beans. These options are the "good carbs" and contain high amounts of fiber, minerals, vitamins, and nutrients to support health in the body and fight disease.

When a whole food is processed and packaged it loses a lot of its fiber and nutrients, and is accompanied by additives, preservatives, and chemicals that support illness in the body; we often hear this type of food termed an "empty calorie" food because it really doesn't provide the body anything in the way of nourishment. These are considered "bad carbs." These processed food products also create imbalances in our blood sugar, while the whole food options help our blood sugar remain steady. Balanced blood sugar means a healthy body, minimal inflammation, and good energy.

Protein

Protein is found all throughout our body; in muscle, bone, skin, hair, and virtually every other body part or tissue. It makes up the enzymes that power many chemical reactions and the hemoglobin that carries oxygen in your blood. Protein helps to repair muscle and provides sustainable energy for the body.

Protein sources include:

- Beans, nuts, and seeds
- Eggs
- Tofu
- Bison, beef, and pork
- Chicken and turkey
- Fish and seafood
- Game meat

Listen to your body and select protein sources that suit you best. Some people do well on a vegetarian diet, while others thrive with some animal protein included in their diet. If you're constantly feeling low on energy or take a while to recover from activity you'll want to explore your protein needs and make sure you're providing your body an adequate amount.

In general, you'll feed the body around 20-30% of your calories with protein. You know your body best, so listen to it well and adjust this need as necessary.

Fat

Essential Fatty Acids are called "essential" for two reasons. First, the body needs healthy fat in order to function properly and create long-term health. Second, it is essential that you consume these fats on a regular basis because the body doesn't create them on its own.

Triglycerides, cholesterol, and other essential fatty acids store energy, insulate us and protect our vital organs. They act as messengers, helping proteins do their jobs. They also start chemical reactions that help control growth, immune function, reproduction, and other aspects of basic metabolism. Fat also helps provide the body with sustainable energy and supports the function of our brain.

Fats help us store fat-soluble vitamins A, C, E, and K for the body to use. These vitamins are necessary for many functions in the body. If it is your goal to live well, stay at a healthy weight, experience good daily energy and be active, you need good fat! Find the types of fat that work best for you and your body.

We often hear about the need to eat Omega 3 fats, but Omega 6 fats are just as important. There is, however, a discrepancy with the ratio of these two fats in our standard American diet. Research suggests that we should consume a ratio of Omega 6:Omega 3 of anywhere from 1:1 to 5:1 in order to be healthy and fight disease in the body. Unfortunately, Americans tend to be at a ratio closer to 20:1! When this ratio is off, and there is an Omega 3 deficiency in the body, you'll experience increased inflammation, depression, weight gain, diabetes, allergies, and even memory problems. This is taking you further away from your long-term health goals! Omega 6 fats will cause inflammation in the body and Omega 3 fats fight inflammation in the body.

It's important to consider the reason for this out-of-balance ratio. Our society largely depends on prepackaged foods for nourishment;

as a whole we're eating crackers, cereal, cookies, salad dressing, and more every day. Most prepackaged goods contain the oils that are high in Omega 6 fats which mean we're subjecting our body to them all the time. And if we're not eating the healthy fats to balance out the Omega 6:Omega 3 ratio, we'll feel the effects of weight gain, inflammation, and the other symptoms I mentioned. While it is important to keep a balanced ratio, it may also seem daunting. Here are some very easy steps you can take to create health in the body and keep your essential fatty acids in check:

Omega 6 fats are prominently found in oils such as: vegetable oil, corn oil, soybean oil, margarine and shortening. Avoid all of these and replace them with high quality oils.

High quality oils include:
- Extra virgin olive oil
- Coconut oil
- Avocado oil

When selecting oils, buy the highest-quality organic products you can afford, since cooking oils are the backbone of so many dishes. Avocado oil and coconut oil have a higher smoke point which will allow you to use them for higher heat cooking. Olive oil should be used at a medium heat and is great addition to salads, dips, and dressings. Good words to look for on the label are organic, first-pressed, cold-pressed, extra-virgin, and unrefined. Words to avoid include expeller-pressed, refined, and solvent extracted.

Vegetable oil, corn oil, soybean oil, and shortening are used in many processed foods including cakes, crackers, bread, and salad dressings. Read the ingredient list on every packaged food and avoid these oils as often as possible. While the best choice in this matter would be to omit processed foods from the diet, you may find it challenging to do it all at once. Start incorporating fresh foods as much as possible and be selective about the choices you make with prepackaged items.

Avocado provides the body healthy fat. Add avocado to salads, sandwiches, wraps, smoothies, and dips or just eat the avocado topped with sea salt as an afternoon snack.

Include raw nuts and seeds in your daily diet: organic flax seeds, chia seeds, sunflower seeds, pumpkin seeds, almonds, and English walnuts all contain healthy fat.

Include wild-caught salmon into your weekly meal planning. You should consume at least two servings of fish per week in addition to any plant-based foods rich in Omega 3.

Eat the whole egg! Egg yolks from pastured hens contain rich Omega 3 fats.

Avoid all oils that have been "hydrogenated" or "partially hydrogenated." You'll find these words in the ingredient list of the oil or packaged food.

Take one step at a time to be rid of the old, inflammatory oils and bring in the new. Do your homework while grocery shopping, read labels, and remove foods that are creating disease in the body instead of feeding your health. You are your best advocate!

How Much Should I Eat of All this Good Stuff?

National Academies Institute of Medicine suggests the following guidelines:

- To meet the body's daily nutritional needs while minimizing risk for chronic disease, adults should get 45% to 65% of their calories from carbohydrates, 20% to 35% from fat, and 10% to 35% from protein.
- There is only one way to get fiber—eat plant foods. Plants such as fruits and vegetables are quality carbohydrates that are loaded with fiber. Studies show an increased risk for

heart disease with low-fiber diets. There is also some evidence to suggest that fiber in the diet may help to prevent colon cancer and promote weight control.

The recommendations:

- Men aged 50 or younger should get 38 grams of fiber a day.
- Women aged 50 or younger should get 25 grams of fiber a day.
- Because we need fewer calories and food as we get older, men over aged 50 should get 30 grams of fiber a day.
- Women over aged 50 should get 21 grams of fiber a day.

Now back to our discussion about calories...

Calories

True or False: All calories are equal.

This seems a trick question! When you look at the definition of a calorie the dictionary will tell us that it is a unit equal to the kilocalorie, used to express the heat output of an organism and the fuel or energy value of food. This would lead us to believe that all calories are then equal, because regardless of where each calorie comes from, it provides us a unit of energy.

On the flip side of that (I always enjoy being the devil's advocate) the quality of a calorie can be drastically different. Let's take a look.

200-Calorie Comparisons

You can eat an Original Glaze Krispy Kreme doughnut for 200 calories.

OR

For the same 200 calories you could sauté the following list of vegetables and enjoy as part of your meal:

½ cup tomatoes

½ cup bell peppers

½ cup spinach

½ cup mushrooms

½ cup broccoli

½ cup asparagus

½ cup onion

½ cup carrots

½ cup cauliflower

That's right, for 200 calories you get the whole list of vegetables, that's 4 ½ cups of goodness!

It is more important to think of the quality of your calories versus just worrying about calorie consumption. If you choose the 4 ½ cups of vegetables you're not only receiving the 200 calories you desire for energy but you're filling your body with antioxidants, vitamins and minerals, and phytonutrients to fight disease and keep you healthy!

The Krispy Kreme doughnut is void of antioxidants, lacks vitamins and minerals and is high in trans fat and sugar. This food product will disrupt your system and feed disease in the body.

While it is important to consider calories in versus calories out for weight loss and weight management, it is even more important to make sure the fuel you put in your body comes from nutrient-dense whole foods. It would be pretty challenging for anyone to eat 4 ½ cups of vegetables in one sitting because there would be too much volume, compared to our ability to eat the Krispy Kreme in a few minutes. Outside of a check-in here and there, I am not a believer of calorie-counting and would rather have you focus on giving your body the right fuel for best success. When you live this way, you will have a healthy relationship with food, without restriction.

Life is full of choices and we cannot expect ourselves to be perfect 100% of the time. My hope for you is that you choose wisely 80% of the time (or more); eating plant-based, nutrient-dense foods so you can soak up all the health benefits and feel well. For the other 20% of the time, enjoy a special treat if you desire...of course, try to choose a whole food treat to avoid trans fats and large amounts of sugar.

So is the answer to the question TRUE or FALSE? Are all calories created equal? I'll leave it up to you to decide.

✳ EXERCISE: *Calories and Me*

What does your relationship with calories look like?

_____

_____

_____

_____

_____

_____

Calories can often be the restrictive, manipulative one in the relationship; do you find this to be true? If so, how?

_____

_____

_____

_____

_____

_____

Have you broken off your relationship with calories? How do you feel as a result?

If you haven't yet divorced yourself from calorie counting, how do you think it would serve you to do so?

In this journey, you're going to find yourself growing a lot, expanding your knowledge and finding ways to incorporate new strategies to build health and happiness. Be open to this learning process, and know that there are many good changes to come!

We all tend to do what we know, not even realizing sometimes there are unintended consequences as a result. The coolest part of all of this is that we are constantly learning, and implementing new healthy habits. I'm thrilled to support you in this journey. You rock!

CHAPTER 13

Meal Prep and Planning

There's one question I get asked often when it comes to lunches and meal making and that is: "How can my family eat healthy meals when I have no time to cook?"

I'm in the same boat as many of you, working full time, caring for children and their activities, and taking care of many other household duties too. There's often very little time in the day to make it all happen so the key to success begins with one vital task... PREPARATION. This is also true if you're working through a health crisis. In the lowest point of my illness, I functioned only 20 to 30 minutes a day at increments of 5-10 minutes of standing. Sometimes we have to get creative with our plan:

- While it's always best to purchase fresh produce, and chop the produce yourself, you can opt for the prechopped vegetable, fruit, and leafy green packs to create ease in your life.
- Have the family pitch in as much as possible and if you have a friend or loved one who enjoys to cook, invite them over to do a freezer meal frenzy! My friend Jess and I would do this. We'd each find three recipes and buy enough ingredients for two families. She'd come to my home, and we'd prep all the food as a team and then create the freezer meals for future

use. While it was a longer day of preparation, I would love this time together and the fact that my freezer would be full with six meals!

- If needed you can purchase prepared or prepackaged food such as organic sausages, homemade soups from the soup bar at the grocery store, or salad fixings for quick and easy dinners.
- Serve a hearty sandwich and add raw veggies and dip for an added boost of nutrients.
- If your body needs extra rest, don't be shy about asking a friend to create a meal train for you. Friends, loved ones and neighbors alike enjoy helping one another out; let them know you're in need.

Meals don't have to be gourmet and fancy, they just need to get the job done. Nourishment is the key.

Think about any big accomplishment you've experienced. How did you get there? My assumption is that it took planning and preparation to make it happen. Healthy eating requires the same planning and preparation as any other goal you've set for yourself. It's a huge accomplishment to consistently serve your family healthy, nourishing meals. Here's the secret to making it happen...

Involve the family when creating your shopping list. Ask everyone which vegetables they'd like to see included in meals for the week. Also ask them what one new vegetable they want to try. If possible, take your children along to the grocery store; teach them how to select good produce and how to identify an organic piece of produce versus conventional. The more they can get their senses involved, the easier your sales job is when it's time to take a bite.

Create your meal plan for the week. Find a quiet moment of time each week to sit down and plan your weekly menu; include breakfast, lunch and dinners.

- Here's a snapshot of a weekly menu from our house:

	Monday	Tuesday	Wednesday	Thursday	Friday	Saturday	Sunday
Breakfast	Veg scramble	Baked oatmeal, berry smoothie	Yogurt parfait (goat yogurt, nut granola, berries)	Breakfast burritos, berries	Apple Pie Oatmeal	Free for all	Homemade oat pancakes, bacon
Lunch	Veg soup, crackers, clementine	Turkey lettuce wraps, apples, veg sticks	Brown rice bowls, pears	Quinoa salad, cheese slices, grapes, veg sticks	Spaghetti, peas, fruit salad	Leftovers, clean out the fridge!	Free for all
Dinner	Salmon, asparagus, quinoa & spinach salad	Brown rice bowls	Veg soup, ½ panini, green smoothie	Spaghetti, broccoli	Turkey burgers, homemade fries, shakes	Homemade BBQ chicken pizza, salad	Black bean chili, corn bread

Please notice that I'm using a few items in repetition throughout the week. I always have eggs, leafy greens, vegetables, fruit, oats, brown rice, quinoa, beans, greens, crackers, yogurt, and various meats on hand so I can create a meal in quick fashion. If you stock your pantry with the necessities, you can create a meal anytime.

Select a day to shop and prep. Schedule a 2.5 hour window so you may complete your grocery shopping and then come home and clean and prep all your vegetables.

Purchase a vegetable crisper to house all your prepped vegetables. Wash, peel if needed, and chop your veggies into snack size bites. When it's time to use them in a recipe, you only have a couple more cuts to make and you can throw them in the pan.

I do not prep my greens ahead of time unless I have time to wash them and let them completely air dry before refrigerating them. If needed, you can store your greens in a plastic shopping bag with a paper towel inserted into the bag to soak up moisture after washing them. Berries should not be washed until you're ready to eat them, so only wash what you need at the time.

Choose a night on the weekend to soak your beans and brown rice in preparation to cook the next day. Or you can opt to soak them during the day while you're off at work. Beans and brown rice should both soak for eight hours, then be rinsed before cooking. This will aid in your ability to digest beans and for the brown rice, the soaking process removes phytic acid which is naturally occuring in the rice, but not so healthy for us to consume.

After eight hours of overnight soaking, I cook a large 8-10 serving pot of rice to be used for the week ahead.

After eight hours of soaking, I'll cook my beans on the stove top or pop them into the crockpot on low to cook throughout the day (I do add water of course). They'll be ready for my meals in the week ahead and while the beans are cooking I can be prepping other meals.

Do as much as possible during your sheduled prep time to create marinades, make soups, prep vegetables, and possibly even cook some of the vegetables you'll need. I often will roast two large cookie sheets of vegetables. I then use these in the breakfast scramble, breakfast burrito, brown rice bowl, and on top of a salad. While my beans and rice are cooking away I'll make one or two pots of soup and make sure any sauces or marinades are prepared. Before the afternoon is done, I have soup, veggies, sauces, beans, and rice all ready to go. My week ahead will be an easy one!

Sometimes I make a double recipe of a meal that will freeze well. We eat one meal for dinner and I'll freeze the other for an easy go-to meal for the weeks ahead. This is very easy to do with soup recipes.

By following these simple rules, you free up time throughout the week which can be dedicated to self-care, fun, relationships, or time to simply relax. The choice is yours. Know that it's possible to make healthy meals in 15-20 minutes every night when you've taken the steps to prepare ahead of time. Get the family involved, have fun with the planning (kids love backwards day when we have breakfast for dinner...let them plan a day of meals with you too!), and feel blessed to be able to share this act of kindness with your loved ones. You're providing nourishment that extends far beyond the food on their plate.

Healthy Shopping on a Budget

Budgeting is a practice that we implement in many areas of our life: we budget our money, our time, and our efforts. For if we didn't, we may end up broke, burned out and exhausted! Often, the act of creating a budget and living within our means involves making choices that support us in our decision to save. The practice of shopping on a budget is no different. In order to achieve your goals, you'll need to make choices that support you in doing so.

Shop on a Budget and Still Eat Healthy Nourishing Foods by Following These Tips:

1. Decide to make healthy shopping part of your lifestyle; dedicate the time and effort needed to sort out your personal budget and plan accordingly. Once you get your feet wet and complete a few shopping trips, you'll better understand how to meet the needs of your family while achieving your money goals.

2. Plan ahead. A budget-conscious shopper has a plan in place. While there are a few coupons available for whole, fresh foods, you can still be strategic by reviewing the sale items and planning your weekly menu accordingly.

3. Avoid shopping in the aisles of the grocery store and fill up on the produce section of the store.

4. When possible, purchase non-perishable items in bulk for cost savings. Warehouses such as Costco and Sam's Club allow you to do so as well as online stores such as amazon.com.

5. Decide what your priorities are; use the "wants versus needs" exercise to help you out. If you're struggling to prioritize where you spend your money, you can begin by asking yourself if the item is a "want" or "need" in your life. If it's a "need," then it must be a priority. This means that you may have to give up purchasing the $100 pair of shoes to achieve your goals and include all of your needs into your lifestyle.

6. For every meal, fill your plate with 80% plant-based foods: vegetables, fruit, whole grains, beans, leafy greens, nuts and seeds. The other 20% of the meal may include organic animal products such as meat, dairy, and eggs. This will help you gain a lot of nourishment while staying on budget.

7. Instead of purchasing boxed snacks, cookies, and chips, take the opportunity to schedule one or two afternoons a month where you can bake your own goods and freeze for future consumption.

8. It's always a fun and healthy treat to buy locally. Check into the option of a CSA (Community Supported Agriculture) or door-to-door organics company to deliver fresh fruit and vegetables. These options can provide a cost savings in the long run. Shopping at local farmer's markets can also help you save some pennies.

9. Stock your pantry and refrigerator with cost-effective staples (see below).

10. Remember that convenience doesn't always come without consequence. Making the investment in your health today means less money being given to doctors, hospitals, and pharmaceutical companies later on. Whole, fresh foods will nourish your body and fight disease so you may enjoy all your days for the long haul. That's a "need" in my book, how about yours?

In order to be a savvy shopper, you'll want to focus on whole foods that you can purchase in bulk. The examples below will help outline what it would cost on a per serving basis to purchase a bag of rice or oats, for example. If you take the example of oats, it is much more cost effective to have this staple in your pantry in bulk, than to buy the instant packets of oatmeal that tend to contain a lot of sugar and added flavoring. You can spend $0.36 on one serving of oatmeal from your bulk purchase and add the sweetener and fruit of your choice to it. This creates not only a healthier option, but saves you money.

Cost Effective Pantry Staples:

Brown Rice: $0.16 per serving

Oats: $0.36 per serving

Quinoa: $0.63 per serving

Black Beans (or any other type of bean):

    Can of beans: $0.26 per serving

    Bag of dry beans: $0.17 per serving

Popcorn (organic, non-GMO): $0.21 per serving

Raw Nuts/Seeds:

    Raw Almonds: $0.35 per serving

    Raw Walnuts or Pecans: $0.48 per serving

Organic Whole Wheat Flour: 5 lb. bag is $3.98

Almond Meal: 6 lb. bag is $16.49 for GF baking

Coconut Oil: $0.23 per tablespoon

You'll also want to stock up on produce to ensure you're getting as many disease-fighting nutrients as possible every day. You can add them to prepackaged foods such as spaghetti sauce, organic sausage, or add them to brown rice and beans for a well-rounded meal.

Fruits, Leafy Greens, and Vegetables

The savvy shopper will select produce items that are on sale and couple the lower-priced items with some higher-priced counterparts. For example, you could add onion, kale, garlic, and bell peppers to a spaghetti sauce. The kale, onion and garlic are inexpensive items while the organic peppers will run you about $3.50 per pound. In total though, you're paying very little to add nutrients to your meal and the sum of the vegetables provides you a large portion for feeding the whole family.

Challenge yourself to see how many fruits and vegetables you can fit into your shopping cart for $75.00; I think you'll be amazed with the results!

Using staples that are versatile, plant-based, and full of fiber and nutrients will keep you satiated and on top of your game whether you're headed off to work, school, or play.

CHAPTER 14

What's in a Name?

Now that you know how to shop on a budget, it's time to learn the importance of detective work. Grocery shopping today is like sending an undercover detective into the streets to find the criminal. As unfortunate as it is, you must advocate for yourself and do investigative work every time you shop. In this chapter you'll learn how to find the truth in every food product, and how to select the best fresh produce for you and the family. Grab your spy gear; it's time to go undercover!

Go Organic

While it's best to eat organically for long-term health, there are some fruits and vegetables deemed safe from the Environmental Working Group (EWG) to be purchased as conventional produce. Conventional produce refers to produce that is not grown organically, and pesticides are used in the growing process.

A Quick Tip on How to Identify Organic Produce:

Every piece of produce contains a PLU code that will help you identify whether the food is organic, or conventionally grown. No more need to wonder what's what, here's the scoop on PLU codes:

Understanding PLU Codes

Conventional Produce

4-digit number within the 3000 or 4000 series

Pesticides are used. Could potentially be a Genetically Modified Organism (GMO)

Pesticide exposure has been associated with cancer as well as negative neurological, reproductive and fertility outcomes.

Be selective and refer to the Clean 15 list at www.ewg.org

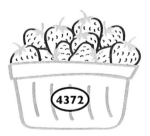

4372

Organic Produce

5-digit number that begins with the number 9

Organically grown without the use of pesticides

The use of Genetically Modified Organisms (GMOs) is prohibited in organic products.

Select products labeled "100% Organic" "USDA Organic" or "Certified Organic" when possible.

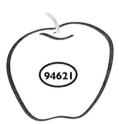

94621

GMO Produce

5-digit number beginning with the prefix "8" was being reserved for GMO Products

However, the "8" prefix was never used at retail. They are stripping this "8" prefix of the GMO designation and will use it elsewhere in the future.

There is NO current PLU code labeling for GMO products.

Look for the following label on the food packages. For a full list of Non-GMO Project Verified products, please visit livingnongmo.org

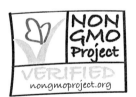

NON GMO Project VERIFIED
nongmoproject.org

The Clean Fifteen and the Dirty Dozen

The Clean Fifteen list I share below is provided by EWG and identifies the produce that has the least amount of pesticides. If organic options are not available for the foods on this list, you can feel confident purchasing them in conventional form. The Dirty Dozen, on the other hand, are the fruits, vegetables, and leafy greens that contain the largest amounts of pesticides and can be harmful to the body in their conventional form. The items listed in the Dirty Dozen should be purchased organically to achieve optimal health.

Life doesn't always allow for organic food to be available; we dine out at restaurants, eat at friends' homes, and travel through airports. The key is to do the best you can with what you're provided. In the end, it's necessary that you get the fruits, vegetables, and greens into your diet and a conventional option will be better than no option at all. Fill your plate with color and enjoy all the robust flavors of these foods!

The Clean Fifteen

- Asparagus
- Avocados
- Cabbage
- Cantaloupe
- Cauliflower
- Eggplant
- Grapefruit
- Kiwi
- Mangoes
- Onions
- Papayas
- Pineapples
- Sweet corn
- Frozen sweet peas
- Sweet potatoes

Dirty Dozen

- Apples
- Celery
- Cherry tomatoes
- Cucumbers
- Grapes
- Nectarines

- Peaches
- Potatoes
- Snap peas
- Spinach
- Strawberries
- Sweet bell peppers

Plus hot peppers, kale, and collard greens.

The question always comes up, "Is it worth it to buy organic?" My answer is, "How could it not be?" Pesticide use has been linked to various cancers, birth defects, learning disabilities, and more. In addition to this, thousands of people visit the hospital every year due to pesticide poisoning.

The goal of using these chemicals is to kill off insects and preserve the crop. With enough repetitive exposure it's not too far fetched to think that they could be killing us too!

While some organic produce can be more expensive than its conventional counterpart I encourage you to think of the long-term cost savings you provide you and your family by purchasing organic produce. Proactive health care is far less expensive than hospital bills, doctor visits, and disease management. You may want to explore giving up something in one area of your life to have the means to purchase organic food. As a family, we often shop at consignment shops, and use gift cards we've received from holidays to purchase larger ticket items. Eating organically has become a way of life for my family, but we've needed to make shifts elsewhere to create this lifestyle. Identify what's most important for you and your loved ones. Decide on ways to save elsewhere to achieve your goals, be selective about what you purchase organically versus conventionally, and do your best with what you have.

EWG is an amazing non-profit organization which supports the community to achieve healthy living. You can explore their website to find information on various toxins, and feel empowered to make the best decisions for you and your family.

Read Labels!

Do you remember this commercial that came out a few years ago? It was for a yogurt that was packaged in a portable tube and glowed in the dark! Just as the commercial suggested, it was like the glow-in-the-dark light saber used in the Star Wars movies. My son, who was about five at the time, begged and begged for me to buy that yogurt…"It's so cool, mom! We have to get it!" he'd say.

My kids fall for just about any marketing you provide them; cartoon characters, strong looking athletes, happy smiles, contests. As much as I hate to say it, adults aren't too far off from the kids. We'll look at the front panel of a packaged food item and assume from the photos, key messages, and beautiful layout that it could be a healthy option. However, the front of the food package is simply a commercial and largely the food maker's marketing campaign. You've got to take a deeper look into the truth of the matter, and do your investigative work.

Back to the glow-in-the-dark yogurt…I asked my son, "What do you think they use to make the color of the yogurt green, is it asparagus, broccoli, or maybe green beans?" While he didn't know the answer, he knew enough that it wasn't coming from a vegetable. He also knew at the young age of five that there wasn't any food he'd ever eaten that glowed in the dark. This was the beginning of many conversations with him and my daughter around the need to do investigative work with the food in our environment. There's a difference between "whole food" that comes from our earth and "food products" that are created in manufacturing plants and laboratories.

Take time to know where your food comes from; if it doesn't come from the earth then read the ingredient list to assess the quality of the ingredients you're consuming. Most processed foods contain multiple sugars, food coloring, added preservatives, and even cancer-causing chemicals.

As Michael Pollan shared with us in *The Omnivore's Dilemma*, if you can't read it, pronounce it or understand it, do NOT put it in your body. It's as simple as that. When selecting a packaged food, select only those with whole ingredients, and stick to an ingredient list that is five ingredients or less. You'll feel better and your body will thank you for it!

Rules for Reading Labels

The front of the box is the commercial; do not trust what you see. Locate the nutrition label and ingredient list on the side or back of the box.

Check the serving size listed at the top of the nutrition label. This is important because we tend to eat much larger portions than the food companies offer as a serving size. If you're eating double the serving size, you then need to double the grams of fiber, sugar, carbohydrates, etc. from the rest of the nutrition panel.

Peek at the grams of fiber per serving. The food product should contain at least 2 grams (preferably more) of fiber per 100 calories. Two grams of fiber per 100 calories is a good indication you're getting a whole grain food product.

Peek at the grams of sugar per serving. It is best to avoid processed sugar. Keep consumption of added sugar to 25 grams or less per day. As stated above, be sure to note the serving size for the grams of sugar. Most often you're probably consuming two to three times the indicated serving size, therefore consuming more sugar than listed.

Be aware of trans fats. This type of fat is very unhealthy for the body and should be avoided. Food companies have the opportunity to play a few tricks with serving size and trans fats. If they can keep the trans fat content of a serving size to less than .5 grams, they can list it as "0" in that food product. This is a problem for multiple reasons: first, we most likely will eat more than one serving size, therefore consuming harmful amounts of trans fat. Second, it allows the nutrition facts to be manipulated in such a way that if your investigative work ends there, you'll never realize you're consuming trans fats at all. This leads us to the next rule for reading labels…

The Truth Lies Beyond the Nutrition Facts

The truth lies in one, and only one, place on any food packaging and that is in the ingredient list.

The ingredient list contains the ingredients of the food product, listed from the largest ingredients to the smallest ingredients. It can be an eye-opening experience to navigate an ingredient list, only to find out that the food product you thought was fresh and whole, contains close to 50 ingredients, or is full of preservatives and words you've never heard before. I can't tell you how many times this happened early on in my health journey.

Take note of how many forms of sugar you find in an ingredient list.

Look to see if the food company is using healthy fats in their food product, or a highly inflammatory one. Or even one that contains trans fats! This, by the way, is the one way to find out if a food contains trans fat; the ingredient list does not lie. Anytime you see the words "hydrogenated vegetable oil," "partially hydrogenated vegetable oil," or "shortening" you'll know that food item contains trans fats.

Beware of the words "natural flavoring." It's difficult to know what is actually in this ingredient mixture and we're constantly exposed to it because it's found in almost every processed food.

Do not eat anything you cannot read, pronounce, or understand.

Focus on at least 80% of your food coming from whole, fresh, colorful foods from the earth; these are the foods that will advocate for your health, provide you disease-fighting phytonutrients and keep you healthy for the long haul.

When you do need to reach for a packaged food to help out in a pinch, be sure to select food items with five or less ingredients. Select organic fare as often as possible, and use these foods to compliment your meal of hearty, colorful whole foods instead of having them be the star of the show.

When selecting a processed meat to add to your meal, be sure to select only uncured, nitrite- and nitrate-free products. If you shop at Whole Foods, your selection will be easy as this is the only type of processed meat they carry! As often as possible, use fresh organic meat and wild caught fish for meal making.

Remember that these prepackaged foods should not be used as a staple in your diet. When you eat these items, it replaces the opportunity to eat whole, fresh foods filled with nutrients, vitamins, and minerals. Be selective about the quality of the prepackaged food you consume, as well as how often you consume them. When consumed occasionally in small amounts, you'll live healthy and be well.

Becoming comfortable with label reading and moving towards organic produce are steps that will pay huge dividends in your journey. It can be a tedious process at the start, and add a bit of time to your shopping trip, but once you do a solid round of label reading and identifying foods that will serve you best, you'll know which foods to reach for, and which ones to leave on the shelf. Even after reading labels for the past seven years, I find surprises. You'll be amazed (and maybe even disgusted) with your discoveries.

Reading Labels

Nutrition Facts

Serving Size 1/2 cup
Servings Per Container 8

Amount Per Serving	
Calories 160 **Calories from fat** 40	
	% Daily Value
Total Fat 5g	8%
Saturated Fat 5g	
Trans Fat 0g	
Cholesterol 0mg	0%
Sodium 230mg	10%
Potassium 95mg	3%
Total Carbohydrate 22g	7%
Dietary Fiber 1g	
Sugars 12g	
Protein 1g	2%
Vitamin A 0% Vitamin C 1%	
Calcium 3% Iron 6%	

Start with the serving size. We most often eat more than one serving of any food. This could make a big difference in trans fats, sugar and more!

Do not worry so much about calories, but rather the quality of your food. Read the Ingredient list!

Read the ingredient list to know if this is good, healthy fat or not.

The FDA states that if trans fat is <.5g/100 cal, companies can label it as 0 grams of trans fat. Check the ingredient list! Anything that says partially hydrogenated or hydrogenated is a trans fat.

Look for foods that contain ≥2 g of fiber per 100 calories. This indicates it's a whole grain food.

KNOW YOUR SERVING SIZE: This is grams of sugar per serving. If you eat 2 servings you'll be close to the recommended limit of 25 g of processed sugar per day!

The Truth Lies in the Ingredients!

Ingredients are listed from largest amount to smallest amount.

Select foods with a short ingredient list, 5 or fewer ingredients

heck to see how any forms of ugar are on the list.

e want high quality gredients!

No High Fructose Corn Syrup

No Preservatives

No Artificial Sweeteners

Ingredients: Enriched Wheat Flour, Corn Flour, High Fructose Corn Syrup, Partially Hydrogenated Vegetable Oil, Sugar, Whole Grain Oat Flour, Salt, Sucralose, Natural Flavor, Yellow 5, Bht to preserve freshness.

Do you see suspicious ingredients? Don't eat anything you:
• Don't Understand
• Can't Pronounce
• Can't read

This product contains trans fat even though it states 0g in the nutrition facts.

CHAPTER **15**

Mindfulness and Food

W e hear about practicing mindfulness in life; taking time to slow down and smell the roses will help all of us reduce stress. This thoughtful approach to life also needs to be practiced at the table. Mindful eating and drinking is as valuable to your health as selecting organic produce and reading labels! Not only will it slow you down so you can enjoy all the flavors, it helps you build awareness and honor your body when it's full.

Practicing mindfulness wasn't something I picked up in my childhood, but I did learn to slow down and practice it in my adult years. Growing up as the oldest of four there were plenty of times I would rush through my meal in hopes of getting seconds from the bowl of mashed potatoes. We were also on the go a lot with all of us playing sports, taking piano lessons and meeting up with friends. Mom and dad did a good job of trying to have family dinners when possible, but we often rotated through the dinner table between our scheduled practices and games. We would chow down and hit the road.

Becoming more mindful has taken a lot of intentional effort and practice. What I do know is that in order to achieve optimal health, we need to pause and be mindful of our actions, including the time spent eating meals.

Essential Digestion...It Starts with Chewing!

When it comes to increased health, it's not just what we eat but how we eat. Digestion actually begins in the mouth, where contact with our teeth and digestive enzymes in our saliva break down food. But these days most of us rush through the whole eating experience, barely acknowledging what we're putting in our mouths. We eat while distracted—working, reading, talking, and watching television—and swallow our food practically whole. On average we chew each bite only eight times. It's no wonder that many people have digestive problems.

There are many great reasons to slow down and chew your food.

- Saliva breaks down food into simple sugars, creating a sweet taste. The more we chew, the sweeter our food becomes, so we don't crave those after-meal sweets.
- Chewing reduces digestive distress and improves assimilation, allowing our bodies to absorb maximum nutrition from each bite of food.
- More chewing produces more endorphins, the brain chemicals responsible for creating good feelings.
- It's also helpful for weight loss, because when we are chewing well, we are more apt to notice when we are full.
- In fact, chewing can promote increased circulation, enhanced immunity, increased energy and endurance, as well as improve skin health and stabilize weight.

- Taking time with a meal, beginning with chewing, allows for enjoyment of the whole experience of eating: the smells, flavors and textures. It helps us to give thanks, to show appreciation for the abundance in our lives and to develop patience and self-control.

The power of chewing is so great that there are stories of concentration camp survivors who, when others could not, made it through with very little food by chewing their meager rations up to 300 times per bite of food. For most of us 300 chews is a daunting and unrealistic goal. However, you can experience the benefits of chewing by increasing to 30 chews per bite. Try it and see how you feel.

Try eating without the TV, computer, smartphone, newspaper or noisy company. Instead pay attention to the food and to how you are breathing and chewing.

This kind of quiet can be disconcerting at first, since we are used to a steady stream of advertising, news, media, email, and demands from others. But as you create a new habit, you will begin to appreciate eating without rushing. You have to eat every day—why not learn to savor and enjoy it?

EXERCISE: *Mindful Eating*

How do you typically eat meals? Are you eating breakfast in the car, lunch at your work desk, and dinner in front of the television? Or do you create a peaceful environment, allowing yourself to be mindful of the food in front of you, the rich flavors on your palate, and the conversations with those around you? Please journal about your eating habits.

What would it provide you to exercise mindfulness at meal time?

Every Process in Your Body Depends on Water... Drink Up!

This may seem like a very basic tip...but necessary! One that every process in your body depends on. The benefits of drinking water extend far beyond quenching your thirst.

Consuming enough water helps maintain balanced bodily fluids. These bodily fluids aid in various processes including digestion, circulation, transportation of nutrients, and the transportation of waste products in and out of cells.

Everyone knows that we should drink eight 8-ounce glasses of water a day. Have you ever wondered if this amount is actually enough? While there's no hard evidence to support this guideline, it is a good place to start. Every person's hydration needs vary; you will be the best judge for the needs of your body system. At a minimum though, everyone should be consuming eight 8-ounce glasses of water per day.

Things to take into consideration when figuring out your daily hydration needs:

EXERCISE: How often do you exercise and release fluids through sweating? It is recommended that you drink water before, during and after any exercise. This will allow you to replenish necessary fluids as you release them.

Environment: Hot and humid environments can increase the release of fluids from your body. This is especially important to consider during travel to hot/humid climates when your body is used to living in a dry environment.

Illness: Flu and cold season wreaks havoc during the winter months. Take extra care to increase your fluids during this time, especially if you're experiencing vomiting or diarrhea which would result in additional loss of fluids.

Pregnancy or Breast Feeding: Large amounts of fluid are used during breast feeding. Be sure to always have water on hand while feeding your infant and hydrate consistently throughout the day.

Signs of a well-hydrated body include odorless urine that is pale yellow in color as well as consistent daily bowel movements.

When the body is lacking fluids your colon will pull fluid from the stool in order to maintain hydration, which leaves you constipated. While talking poo isn't part of everyday conversation, it is a necessary topic to consider. You should have consistent bowel movements; at least once a day if not more. Fiber and fluids are your best combination for daily movement.

I often have clients tell me they drink water when they're thirsty. While this may be a good indication that you need fluids, there is a problem with this plan. Your thirst mechanism goes off when your bodily fluids are low which means you're already behind in fluid consumption. The goal is to stay ahead of the game by hydrating consistently through the day so that you do not feel thirsty.

An easy way to remember to drink water is to drink a glass in the morning, one to two glasses before each meal, a glass between meals and one small glass in the evening before bed. This will only get you to the eight suggested glasses a day, so increase the volume or drink water more often to increase your overall fluid consumption.

Other benefits of drinking enough water include younger looking skin, and better mood. Tufts University researchers found that even mild dehydration is associated with feelings of anger, depression and confusion.

Even though water will not magically wipe away all the wrinkles in the skin, it will plump up your skin and give you a "glowing" appearance when you adequately hydrate. What a great bonus; you can look refreshed and be more productive in work and life just by drinking more water!

The foundation of health begins with our cells. These cells need to be well hydrated and nourished to provide our body and muscles the energy necessary for top performance all day long. When cells don't receive adequate fluid they shrivel up and performance goes down. Muscles fatigue and the body will lack energy. This is a difficult way to function all day, especially when the solution is an easy one.

Along with drinking water, you can count your raw fruits and vegetables as a hydration source. All of these plant foods provide your body structured water which not only nourishes and hydrates the cells in the body, but also provide you disease-fighting antioxidants and healthy fiber.

If plain old water isn't enough excitement for you then try one of these options: brew your own tea, add fruit and herbs to your water, or enjoy hot green or herbal tea for an afternoon treat.

While most liquids hydrate your body I caution you about the amount of sugar you may be consuming. Soda, Gatorade, Vitamin Water, and bottled tea are all options available to us, but the sugar content tends to be very high, and if you opt for the diet-sweetener option you're doing more harm than good to your system. Be creative with various fruits, herbs, and vegetables, and enjoy a spa-like experience all day long.

Be mindful of your choices, while at the table and in life. Take time to ask yourself how your decision will support you in health. Are you giving your body what it needs to be healthy, are you providing your cells the antioxidants and hydration they need to thrive, and do you take time to be present while you dine? Think of the three meals you eat every day and consider your eating habits. Where could you enrich your mindfulness and how would it impact you to do so?

CHAPTER 16

Sugar

Addiction played a major role in my health crisis; there are no two ways about it. The problem was that I never wanted to admit to it. My husband sat me down at two different points and begged me to get the sugary treats out of the house. He would explain that he thought it was contributing to my ill body, and would ask me to change my ways. Bless his heart for trying; I wish I could have been open to hear his words at that time in my life. It had the opposite effect on me; I would rebel every time and eat more and more of the food he wanted me to get rid of. It feels awful even writing it, but it's the truth.

We all do what we know to do. My body knew it loved sugar and the cycle continued for a long period after the interventions. I would try to cut sugar out of the diet, and at one phase in my life I did. Crazy as it may sound, I had withdrawal symptoms just as any addict would. I had cut the sugar cold turkey and I felt like I had the flu, had a horrible headache for days, and was very irritable. It took a great deal of effort to stay sugar free and then we went out to dinner for my birthday.

We were at Bill Knapp's restaurant with my family, a place we frequented growing up. Their chocolate cake was my favorite dessert as a child, and the serving size was large. I ended up ordering a slice for my special day: I ate the whole slice on my own, along with the ice cream, whipped cream, and maraschino cherry that accompanied it. That was the end of the sugar-free road. I was off the wagon again, just like I'd ebbed and flowed so many times before.

Sugar addiction is just as serious as any other, and could arguably be more difficult to kick. Sugar is everywhere in our food system; you can easily find multiple forms of it in processed foods! When I studied as a Certified Health Coach, I learned ways to cut the cravings and naturally ease myself into healthy eating. It's called the crowding out method, and by simply incorporating good food into your diet you will start to naturally remove the sugar-laden ones. It worked beautifully and I've been using it with clients ever since. I still enjoy a piece of dark chocolate most days of the week, but it's a rare occasion you'll see me eating a full dessert. As any addict needs to do, it's best for me to stay away from it all together. Now my husband thinks it's ridiculous when I say I'm craving kale; but it's true! New patterns exist for me now as I continue to learn and improve my health in this journey.

I'll warn you that your relationship with sugar may change after you read through this chapter. It's not your will power or the sugar that's the problem; it's the vicious cycle that exists from the amount of sugar we're consuming. I'm excited to share a few tips with you and hope that someday you connect to tell me you're craving kale too.

The best part of this whole chapter is the sweet treat I share with you at the end; proof you can have your cake and eat it too!

Give Up the Swiss Cake Rolls

Have you thought of a Swiss cake roll while driving down the road, so much so that your mouth begins to salivate and you succumb to the need by pulling directly into the next available gas station to make the purchase? This used to happen to me a lot, and I loved stopping at the gas station because the pack of Swiss cake rolls there included not two, but THREE in the package. Life was excellent and it only took me a few minutes to magically make them all disappear. This was my life as an addict...a sugar addict. As my friend John would say, true story!

Sugar is an addictive substance and we know this for two specific reasons. When you eat sugar, you end up wanting more. And if you ever decide to cut sugar out of your diet cold turkey, as I've had first-hand experience with, you experience withdrawal symptoms; in my case headache, fatigue, moodiness, cravings, and interrupted sleep.

Sugar in its own right is not the cause of the addiction. If we only ate nine pounds of it per year like folks did in the 1800s it wouldn't be an issue. But we are far from that, and most research indicates that we as Americans consume an average of 150 pounds of added sugar per year. This could even be viewed as a conservative number, as others suggest we eat in upwards of 300 pounds of added sugar per year. This level of consumption has sent us into a health crisis.

The average number of items carried in a supermarket in 2014 was 42,214 (Food Marketing Institute). As you can observe when stepping foot into any grocery store, we don't have 42,214 different types of fruits, vegetables, beans, whole grains, and nuts and seeds. Instead, the aisles are filled with prepackaged food products that claim to make our lives easier and are priced effectively to provide convenience. You can even clip coupons for additional savings.

Your savings, however, aren't going to stretch too far; all the forms of sugar, let alone synthetic ingredients like preservatives and food coloring, are going to wreak enough havoc on your system that you'll experience a deterioration of health and eventually it'll mean doctor visits, testing, hospital stays, and other medical bills. No coupons to clip and save for these services.

It takes years for disease to set into the body, and there is consistent research to suggest that sugar feeds disease. How is sugar feeding disease in your body today?

Giving up sugar had been a consistent struggle for me, one that took great effort and attention. As with any addiction, it's best to keep the addictive substance out of reach, away from your home, and avoid social situations that may prompt you to fall back into use. This is not easily accomplished; but you can find a way to do it. Start by cleaning out the house of all forms of processed sugar. Eat something before heading to a party or social event, and if you do decide to eat sugar, consume only a couple of bites and focus on greater fulfillment: the connection with others, the fun you're having dancing to the live band, or the love of learning something new.

Honor the needs of your body, and be selective about the times that you enjoy a couple of bites of a sweet treat. You'll have to do some work with this. Discover what works for you and make the necessary changes to give up the Ding Dongs and Swiss cake rolls. We are all unique and have different needs, but this is one area in which we can all improve. Get rid of the sugar. You'll be richer for it, in health, in finances, and overall happiness.

Steps to Remove Sugar From Your Diet:

1. Reference the Label Reading section of this book in Chapter 14 and read all labels for every prepackaged food product.

2. Clean your pantry, fridge, and freezer of all goods containing any of the common forms of processed sugar: sugar, pure cane sugar, dextrose, sucrose, maltodextrin, corn syrup, high fructose corn syrup, corn syrup solids, maltose, malt syrup, fruit juice, cane juice...the list is even longer so be aware. Anything ending in "ose" indicates it's a form of sugar. When in doubt about any ingredient, you should put the box of food back on the shelf and walk away. Please note that this doesn't mean you should turn to artificial sweeteners; these are a non-negotiable in my book. Artificial sweeteners are made of neurological toxins that can cause more damage than processed sugars.

3. Start filling your body with more naturally sweet foods to lessen the cravings for processed sugar. These foods could include: sweet potatoes, carrots, roasted cauliflower, blueberries, strawberries, peaches, apples, whole grains like brown rice and steel cut oats, nuts and seeds.

4. Use natural sweeteners for all your needs; the benefit to using these natural sweeteners is that most of them are unrefined and therefore contain trace minerals and nutrients. They tend to be lower on the glycemic load which allows for better balanced blood sugar and less cravings.

5. Instead of purchasing prepackaged sweets like cookies, cakes, and breads consider making your own and use the natural sweetener options to do so.

6. We often think of sugary foods as candy and desserts but all the "white foods" contribute just as much to our health crisis. Lower your consumption of these white foods (bagels, bread, pasta, cookies, cakes) in your diet and replace with whole grains such as brown rice, quinoa, millet, amaranth, teff and oats.

7. Fat and fiber are your friends; they each help balance the digestion of sugar so your body stays better balanced. Fill up on high-fiber content foods such as leafy greens, vegetables, beans, and whole grains as well as good fat: salmon, sardines, coconut oil, extra-virgin olive oil, avocado, nuts and seeds.

8. When you experience a craving take a moment to ask yourself these questions:

   • What am I feeling in this moment? (stress, anger, sadness, etc.)

   • Will this food I'm craving truly satiate my need or emotion?

   • How can I best serve the needs of my body?

   By pausing and asking yourself these questions you'll become more aware of the deeper root of your craving and best honor the needs of your body by making a sound, thoughtful decision.

9. There will be moments where you fall off track, or make a decision that you later regret. It happens to all of us. When this takes place I ask that you be very kind and patient with yourself. Explore the reasons you may have made the decision, go back to asking yourself what you were feeling, and assess the situation. We learn from each of our experiences, and this one is no different. It'll help build more awareness and empower you to reach your health goals.

Natural Sweeteners

Natural sweeteners provide us the opportunity to sweeten our food in a more natural, healthy way than the sugar options found in most processed foods. While this approach will benefit our body a bit more than regular old sugar, we must remember that they are all still sweeteners and all sweeteners should be used in moderation in order to reach optimal health.

Below are a few of my favorites.

Agave Nectar: This is a natural liquid sweetener made from the juice of the agave cactus. It is 1.4 times sweeter than refined sugar but has been found to have a lower GI (Glucose Index) score which means less disruption to the body's blood sugar levels.

Note of caution for agave nectar: This sweetener contains high amounts of fructose (even higher than high-fructose corn syrup) and some research suggest that fructose doesn't allow our appetite hormones to shut off, which means that you may end up overeating and decrease your glucose tolerance. As with any sweetener, you'll want to use agave nectar in moderation.

Honey: Honey is one of the oldest sweeteners around and is sweeter than table sugar. It can have a range of flavors from dark and strongly flavored, to light and mildly flavored. Raw honey contains small amounts of enzymes, minerals, and vitamins and has anti-viral, anti-bacterial, and anti-fungal properties. It's also known as a powerful antioxidant, strengthens the immune system, and helps to eliminate allergies when purchased locally in its raw form.

Note of caution for honey: If you have a true sugar addiction and are trying to rid your body of the sugar, you may opt to stay away from honey for a while, as your body tends to respond to honey just as it does sugar. As with all sweeteners, whether you experience sugar addiction or not, honey should be used in moderation.

One of my common medicinal uses for raw honey is to treat skin burns...I've accidentally touched a few hot pot handles in my day! Place raw honey on a Band-Aid and place directly to the burn. The stinging will subside and your skin will heal up nicely!

Maple Syrup: Maple syrup is made from boiled-down maple tree sap and contains many minerals. Be sure you're purchasing 100% maple syrup and not a maple-flavored corn syrup like Log Cabin or Mrs. Butterworth.

Grade B maple syrup is darker in color and contains higher mineral content than Grade A maple syrup and is a nice sweetener for baking and cooking. You may use it to remove the bitter taste from your tomato sauce, add it to your soup to balance out flavor, or use when baking muffins. It's very versatile and a little goes a long way.

Stevia: While the taste of stevia is not a favorite of mine, I often get asked about it. South Americans have used this leafy herb for centuries. It is 100 to 300 times sweeter than white sugar and can be used in cooking and baking. You may find it used in canned/bottled beverages as well. Stevia is a zero calorie food and does not affect blood sugar levels. If you choose to use this sweetener select the green or brown liquid or powders because the white and clear versions are highly refined.

Coconut Palm Sugar (Not to be confused with "palm sugar" –they are two different sweeteners): Coconut palm sugar is low on the glycemic index and higher in nutrients than regular table sugar (which is void of any nutrients). It tastes great and can be used where you use regular sugar for baking and sweetening food in a convenient one-to-one ratio.

The biggest health tip I can provide you around any sweetener is to use all of them in MODERATION. Ideally, you'll get your daily sweets intake through fresh, organic whole foods. When you consume any added sweetener in excess, it can cause a lot of problems like metabolic syndrome, obesity, diabetes, and cardiovascular disease. So do your body a favor and reserve the use of these sweeteners for special treats and occasions.

Uses and Ratios for Natural Sweeteners

Sweetener	Amount = 1 cup sugar	Uses
Honey	1/2 - 2/3 cup	All-purpose
Maple Syrup	1/2 - 3/4 cup	Baking, desserts, sauces
Coconut Palm Sugar	1 cup	All-purpose
Agave Nectar	2/3 cup and reduce other liquids by 1/4 to 1/3 cup	All-purpose

Please consider the fact that sweeteners, regardless of being a natural option or not, are still sweeteners. We should reserve sweets for occasional consumption and fill up on whole forms of sugar like vegetables, fruits and whole grains.

RECIPE: *Decadent Chocolate Cake*
(Gluten, Grain and Yeast Free)

I'd like to share this recipe with you…it's a natural approach to the disease-feeding Swiss cake roll I used to pull into the gas station for. This is a divine dessert sure to please the palate without inspiring cravings.

Ingredients

1 ½ cups dark chocolate, broken into pieces (70% or greater cocoa content)

1 (19 oz) can garbanzo beans, rinsed and drained

4 eggs

¾ cup Organic Coconut Palm Sugar

½ tsp baking powder

1 Tbsp confection's sugar for dusting

Directions

- Preheat oven to 350 ° Fahrenheit.
- Grease a 9-inch round cake pan (or pie pan) with organic butter.
- Place chocolate pieces into a small sauce pan on the stove over medium-low heat. Stir constantly until chocolate is melted into smooth creaminess. Do not leave chocolate unattended; it will burn quickly.
- Pour beans and eggs into a food processor bowl. Process until smooth. Add the coconut palm sugar and baking powder and pulse to blend. Pour in the melted chocolate and blend until smooth.
- Wipe down the sides of the bowl to ensure all chocolate and batter is mixed together. Pulse for final blending.
- Pour batter into prepared cake pan.

- Cook for 40 minutes or until a knife inserted into the center of the cake comes out clean.
- Cool in pan on a wire rack for 15 minutes.
- Run a knife along the edge of the cake pan to loosen the sides of the cake from the pan. Place a serving plate on top of your cake pan. Hold the sides of cake pan and serving plate and turn it over to invert the cake onto the plate.
- You may sprinkle with confectioner's sugar just before serving.

I top the center of the cake with an assortment of fresh berries and serve with freshly whipped organic heavy cream. Divinely delish!

The original recipe is compliments of www.allrecipes.com; I have updated it to align with our healthy eating goals.

One thought to keep in mind about sweeteners and sugar; they're found everywhere in our processed-food-focused country! Do your homework, know how many forms of sugar are in your food, select natural sweeteners as often as possible, and eat sweeteners in moderation. Please remember to avoid all artificial sweeteners as they are neurological toxins and harmful to your health.

CHAPTER **17**

Overcome Cravings with Ease

Cravings aren't always a bad thing; sometimes cravings send a message to your body. For instance, if you find yourself craving kale (yes, as I mentioned earlier, this is possible), it may be that your body needs vitamin C or magnesium. Maybe brown rice is a food that sounds good to you all the time; this may mean your body is enjoying the B vitamins and energy it provides you. When craving salt, it could be that your body wants to balance something sweet you've just eaten. There are many reasons that one may experience cravings. The best thing you can do is tune into the cravings you're having, identify the situation you're in (are you stressed, bored, tired, or maybe truly hungry), and assess what the food provides you once you eat it. Did it actually give you energy, or help you focus on your project? You'll start to build awareness around your patterns, and be able to make change as needed.

As you work to transition yourself out of sugar cravings, there are foods that can help you along the way. Let's review the role of whole grains, fruit and vegetables.

Whole Grains

In addition to using the crowding out method, where you add good, healthy foods into your diet and naturally crowd out the sugary ones, another way to help your body avoid sugar cravings is to proactively eat foods that are slower to digest. The body takes longer time to absorb whole grains, and as a result, you're provided sustained, high-quality energy. Whole grains also contain many nutrients to support your body in health.

Some of my favorites include quinoa, brown rice, oats, buckwheat, and teff. Each of these can be used as a yummy hot breakfast cereal. Quinoa is a wonderful addition to salads, teff can be used to make beautiful gluten free crust, and each can be added to any meal as a side dish.

Quinoa

Quinoa (pronounced keen-wah) is a nutritional powerhouse with ancient origins. It was originally cultivated by the Incas more than 5,000 years ago; they referred to it as the "mother of all grains." It contains all nine essential amino acids, making it a great source of protein for vegetarians. Quinoa is also high in magnesium, fiber, calcium, phosphorus, iron, copper, manganese, riboflavin, and zinc.

While quinoa is widely considered a grain, it's actually the seed of a plant called Chenopodium or Goosefoot, related to chard and spinach. Quinoa is a gluten-free grain and has a similar effect as other whole grains in helping to stabilize blood sugar.

It has a waxy protective coating called saponin, which can leave a bitter taste. For best results, rinse quinoa before you cook it or even soak it for a few minutes and then rinse. I enjoy toasting the rinsed quinoa before adding water to cook. When cooked, it has a fluffy, slightly crunchy texture. Try it in soups, salads, as breakfast porridge or as its own side dish.

For quinoa, and whole grains in general, the majority of digestion occurs in the mouth through chewing and exposure to saliva. For optimal nutrition and assimilation, it is vital to chew your grains well. Make it a habit to chew each bite 20 times or more. See how this simple practice can help your digestion and overall focus for the rest of your day.

Fruits and Vegetables

"An apple a day keeps the doctor away." We've all heard this saying many times in our lives, but do you know why it's true? Let's dig into the reasons why daily fruit and vegetable consumption is necessary for all of us.

Test Your Knowledge:

1. How do you distinguish a fruit from a vegetable?
2. What type of vitamins do we need to replenish every day?
3. How many servings of fruit and vegetables should we consume daily?
4. What is a serving size?
5. Do all fruits contain about the same amount of sugar?

Answer Key:

1. How do you distinguish a fruit from a vegetable?

Fruits contain the seeds that will produce the next generation of plants, which flower and fruit again.

2. What type of vitamins do we need to replenish every day?

We need to replenish our water-soluble vitamins every day. Unlike fat-soluble vitamins, which our bodies store for future use, water-soluble vitamins cannot be stored. In order for our bodies to run at an optimal level, we need to eat fruits and vegetables every day in order to get these water-soluble vitamins. Water-soluble vitamins include vitamin C, the B vitamins and folic acid.

Vitamins are considered "essential" because our bodies cannot produce them, so it is essential that we get them through the foods we eat. Fruits and vegetables contain one of the richest sources of water-soluble vitamins.

As an added bonus, we also get loads of phytonutrients from our fresh produce, which helps fight oxidative stress and disease in the body.

3. **How many servings of fruits and vegetables should we consume daily?**

As a rule of thumb, your vegetable intake should be twice that of your fruit intake. Each of us should be eating 3-4 servings of fruit and 8-9 servings of vegetables every day, seven days a week, in order to achieve proper physiological functioning and optimal health. The body may survive on less for some time, as it takes a while for the effects of vitamin deficiencies to settle into the body. However, the effects of vitamin and nutrient deficiencies cannot be avoided and will appear in the body as fatigue, reduced immune function, and more. Without adequate servings of fruit and vegetables in our diet, we are depriving our body of essential vitamins and nutrients and will not achieve the optimal health we desire.

Remember to eat a variety of colorful fruits and vegetables to offer the body an array of disease-fighting phytonutrients.

4. **What is a serving size?**

In general, a serving size of fruit is ½ cup, or one medium size piece of fruit. Here's a little guide to follow:
- 1 medium pear, apple or orange
- 1 small banana
- ½ cup grapes, strawberries, blueberries

- ½ grapefruit
- 1 cup diced melon
- ¼ cup dried fruit
- ¾ cup juice

In general, a serving of vegetables is 1 cup of leafy greens, or ½ cup of raw chopped vegetables.

In a day's time you should achieve eating 1½-2 cups of fruit per day and 4-4½ cups of vegetables per day. For some, this can seem overwhelming. Take baby steps forward every day and begin by adding one ½ cup serving to your diet. Every few days, continue to add another serving until you reach your daily goal. Your body will thank you for it, your skin will glow, you'll experience more sustainable energy and feel an overall improvement in your health over time.

5. Do all fruits contain about the same amount of sugar?

No. This is especially important for individuals with diabetes or insulin resistance to understand. Fruits are a concentrated source of carbohydrates and/or sugars and each of these foods will affect our blood sugar levels differently. The tool we use to assess how food impacts our blood sugar level is the Glycemic Index (GI). A food's GI is a value that ranks foods based on their immediate effect on blood sugar levels. It is a measure of how much your blood sugar increases over a period of two or three hours after a meal.

Sweet fruits such as pineapple, mango, and papaya break down quickly during digestion and are considered high GI foods. If you consume these fruits with a lower GI food, you'll slow the release of sugar into the bloodstream and create a lower GI effect. Fruits that are lower on the glycemic index include apples, grapefruit, pears, berries, and plums.

The Amazing Avocado

Although many people serve the avocado as a vegetable, it's actually a type of tropical fruit. This versatile food can be used in many ways. Avocados provide the best nutritional content when eaten raw. Add ½ an avocado to your morning smoothie for a rich, creamy texture, chop some up and add it to your afternoon salad, or top a piece of halibut with avocado and tomato for dinner. Even snacks can be provided a boost by mashing the avocado and creating a dip for veggies and more. The most important factor is to get this fabulous food into your diet; it has too many health benefits not to.

Health Benefits of the Avocado

Promotes Heart Health:

- Avocados contain heart-healthy monounsaturated fat which can help lower total cholesterol and LDL cholesterol while improving your HDL cholesterol.
- Potassium is a mineral that helps regulate your blood pressure and avocados are a good source of this mineral.
- Adequate levels of fiber are needed in the body to keep your heart healthy. The avocado contains 7.3 grams in a one-cup serving!
- Avocados are rich in folic acid and vitamin B6 which help promote clean and healthy arteries.

Anti-Inflammatory Benefits:

- The antioxidants along with Omega 3 fatty acids found in avocado help prevent both osteoarthritis and rheumatoid arthritis.

Absorption of Nutrients:

- Carotenoids are antioxidants that protect our cells from free radicals, enhance our immune system, and promote eye and lung health. Many leafy greens and vegetables contain various carotenoids and fat soluble vitamins that provide us health benefits. Fat soluble means that these antioxidants and vitamins must be accompanied by fat to be absorbed by the body. Adding avocado to your salad or sandwich can help you absorb all the nutrients your body needs.

• New research is appearing to suggest that avocado can also help prevent various cancers and help regulate your blood sugar. Adding this good fat to your snacks and meals will boost your health and help you stay trim.

Fun Fact

Avocados do not ripen on the tree. It is only after harvesting that an avocado will fully ripen. It's no wonder we see a lot of hard avocados in the grocery store. A ripened avocado will have skin that is dark green, almost black, in color and will "give" to gentle pressure.

If you're in need of a ripened avocado in quick fashion, you can always place the avocado in a brown paper bag to increase the ripening process. Adding a banana or apple will boost it even more. Just be sure to check on the process frequently, as you don't want an over ripened avocado. Once the avocado is fully ripened you can store it in the refrigerator for two days; this will keep it from ripening further (do not refrigerate unripe avocados as they will never ripen).

There are Many Ways to Slice an Avocado...

But the best way to prepare an avocado is peeling the skin from the flesh. This will ensure you get as much of the dark green flesh which contains the most nutrients as possible. Slice the avocado lengthwise and twist the two sections apart. Remove the center pit with a spoon. Slice each section of the avocado lengthwise one more time so you have four pieces. Pull the skin back from each slice, just as you would peel a banana. Sprinkle with lemon or lime juice to avoid browning. Dice and serve.

Get the Most from Your Fruit

Be sure to eat the skin of your fruit, as this adds an amazing amount of fiber to your meal which will help slow down digestion, and in turn slow the release of sugar into the bloodstream.

Fresh fruit is always best! The GI for fruit juice and dried fruit is much higher than its whole fresh fruit counterpart. Juice contains less pulp and skin than the whole fruit and drying fruit concentrates its sugar content.

While an apple a day will surely help keep the doctor away, it is best to eat a variety of fruit and vegetables. Every different color in your food provides the body a variety of phytonutrients and health benefits.

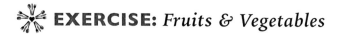 **EXERCISE:** *Fruits & Vegetables*

How many servings of fruit do you consume daily? _____

How many servings of vegetables do you consume daily? _____

What will you do this week to work toward your optimal servings of fruit and vegetables?

_____

_____

_____

_____

CHAPTER **18**

Health Begins in Your Cells

Take care of your body. It's the only place you have to live. ~ Jim Rohn

Getting to the root cause of a problem can be challenging, but is necessary for long-term health. This concept wasn't ever something I considered until after my diagnosis. Once I decided I was going to figure out how to live, I made it my mission to explore every kind of care possible to see if I could find someone to help me. I ventured in and out of many offices, as I had done so many times before, and after a year and three months I found my gal!

She happened to be a chiropractor and functional medicine doctor. At the time, I didn't know exactly what functional medicine meant, but I liked how she navigated my illness and something stood out in our first conversation. I had asked her if she had ever treated anyone with mitochondrial myopathy, and she stated that she doesn't treat a diagnosis, she treats the symptoms. This was my intro into identifying the root cause of the problem.

In all my doctor visits over two years leading up to my diagnosis, I had learned about taking drugs to treat the depression they thought I had, drugs to shut my immune system down for the arthritis, and anti-inflammatory drugs to help when the joint pain was too much to bear. But never once did someone try to explain WHY my immune system may have attacked my body in the first place, or why my cells were damaged and no longer functioning. This doctor was on to something and I was excited about where we were headed.

I had already been supporting my body with whole foods, practicing meditation, and had rid our home of toxins by the time I met my functional medicine doctor. I did feel better as a result of my efforts but was far from being out of the woods. She ran tests and found that I had very high levels of mercury and uranium in my body, a slew of food allergies, and I broke the record for having the highest candida score she had ever seen. Now, this is nothing to celebrate having the highest score and all, but the cause for celebration was the fact that she found missing pieces to the puzzle!

All of the information she gathered helped her treat the root cause of my symptoms and over a period of a couple of years, my cells were healthy and we got my body back to functioning at a good level.

The health of our body begins with the health of our cells. We need to protect them, give them the correct nourishment to thrive, and hydrate them well for peak performance. We're going to dive into oxidative stress, satiating smoothies and super-duper foods to keep your cells happy and strong for the long haul. Roll up your sleeves, grab your highlighter and feel free to write in the margins. Class is in session.

Take Care of Your Cells

Cells are the foundation of health; without them working to their highest potential, we cannot achieve our healthiest body. In order to support our cells, we must nourish them properly through food, hydrate well, and mitigate stress in our life. Cells can easily be compromised from free radicals and oxidative stress. The key to long-term health is understanding how to combat each of these to provide the healthiest environment for our cells to thrive.

I am not a scientist, nor pretend to be. The best way to describe oxidative stress and free radicals to you is to quote Dr. Andrew Weil, MD; he describes it beautifully for all of us to understand. This quote comes from an article he wrote on understanding oxidative stress; you may also read more in his book *Healthy Aging: A Lifelong Guide to Your Physical and Spiritual Well-Being.* Here's how Dr. Weil describes this complex process:

"Oxidation" is the chemist's term for the process of removing electrons from an atom or molecule. The result of this change can be destructive—rusting iron is a familiar result of oxidation. Here, oxygen is the responsible agent, but other oxidizing agents, such as chlorine, can be as harsh.

Although we need oxygen to live, high concentrations of it are actually corrosive and toxic. We obtain energy by burning fuel with oxygen—that is, by combining digested food with oxygen from the air we breathe. This is a controlled metabolic process that, unfortunately, also generates dangerous byproducts. These include free radicals—electronically unstable atoms or molecules capable of stripping electrons from any other molecules they meet in an effort to achieve stability. In their wake they create even more unstable molecules that then attack their neighbors in domino-like chain reactions.

By the time a free radical chain fizzles out, it may have ripped through vital components of cells like a tornado, causing extensive damage, similar to that caused by ionizing radiation.

Oxidative stress is the total burden placed on organisms by the constant production of free radicals in the normal course of metabolism plus whatever other pressures the environment brings to bear (natural and artificial radiation, toxins in air, food and water; and miscellaneous sources of oxidizing activity, such as tobacco smoke).

Our bodies aren't helpless in the face of these assaults. We have defenses against oxidative stress in the form of physical barriers to contain free radicals at their sites of production within cells; enzymes that neutralize dangerously reactive forms of oxygen; substances in our diets (such as vitamin C and vitamin E) that can "quench" free radicals by donating electrons to them and cutting off the chain reactions early in their course; repair mechanisms to take care of oxidative damage to DNA, proteins and membranes; and complex stress responses that include programmed cell suicide if damage is too great.

A good case can be made for the notion that health depends on a balance between oxidative stress and antioxidant defenses. Aging and age-related diseases reflect the inability of our antioxidant defenses to cope with oxidative stress over time. The good news is that with strong antioxidant defenses, long life without disease should be possible.

The best way to reduce oxidative stress and kill free radicals in our body is to eat whole, nutrient-rich foods. This means we must focus on whole plant foods that contain high amounts of phytonutrients, antioxidants, vitamins, and minerals that proactively fight disease and help heal current health issues.

In this section, we'll explore some of the healthiest common-day foods you can begin incorporating into your diet. Along with reducing oxidative stress, these foods fight disease, increase energy, help you achieve and maintain a healthy weight, and support heart health to name just a few.

Foods to Boost Your Health

Eat Your Greens

As of late, leafy greens have been taking center stage and for very good reason! They are one of the most missed foods in the American diet. These little leaves of green are a powerhouse food and sure to boost your health when consumed daily.

Health benefits of leafy greens include: cardiovascular protection, cholesterol-reduction, cancer prevention, calcium, magnesium, vitamin K, vitamin A, vitamin C, vitamin E, healthy skin, eye protection, and more. They support your upper respiratory system and will aid your immune system in fighting off the common cold.

Let's cover just a few of the options you have available to you. Beyond spinach, broccoli, and kale, you can explore many others! Try bok choy, romaine, spring mix, baby kale, arugula, beet greens, and Swiss chard. For optimal health, remember to rotate your greens and try something new each week.

Spinach

Calorie for calorie, leafy green vegetables like spinach, kale, and broccoli are some of the most nutrient-dense foods you can eat. Spinach happens to have a lighter, sweeter leaf than some of its leafy counterparts and while they all provide high amounts of vitamins, minerals, and antioxidants, spinach takes top rank in a couple of areas.

The health of our gut is important for overall health in our body; new research suggests that spinach contains a key nutrient that protects our digestive tract and minimizes inflammation. This nutrient is called glycoglycerolipids; it is necessary for the plant's photosynthesis and helps protect the lining of our digestive tract from damage.

While many vegetables help aid in cancer prevention, spinach has been the only one to show evidence of protection against aggressive prostate cancer. Researchers haven't identified the specific nutrients that allow for this to occur, but we know that spinach does contain two anti-cancer carotenoids that may contribute to this finding. Beyond prostate cancer, researchers have identified over a dozen different flavonoid compounds in spinach that function as anti-inflammatory and anti-cancer agents. Scientists have even taken some of these flavonoids to create spinach extracts to treat stomach cancer, skin cancer, and breast cancer in laboratory studies. In each scenario, the extracts help slow the progression of the cancer. The amazing powers of whole foods are always at work for our benefit.

Vitamin C will help keep us healthy through the cold and flu season by boosting our immune system. The spinach leaves that are brighter and richer in color and look most "alive" are going to give you the most robust amount of vitamin C. For this reason, avoid those that are yellowish in color, or are looking wilted or old.

Spinach is full of vitamin K; its kale counterpart is the only leafy green to supersede it in rank for containing the most amount of vitamin K per serving. Our bone health depends on vitamin K! (Note: if you are on a blood thinner medication it is important to discuss vitamin K consumption with your doctor and be sure to keep your consumption of leafy greens consistent from day to day.)

One note of caution to be aware of with spinach is that it does contain measurable amounts of oxalates. Oxalates are naturally occurring substances found in plants, animals, and human beings. The problem that can occur with oxalates is that when they become too concentrated in body fluids, they can crystalize and cause health problems. For many, this is not an issue, but for individuals with an existing and untreated kidney or gallbladder problem, it may exacerbate the health condition. For these individuals, it may be best to avoid spinach and select other leafy greens instead.

Laboratory studies have also shown that oxalates may interfere with calcium absorption. It is not clear how much interference takes place, so take the high road and rotate your greens daily incorporating spinach into the mix 1-2 times per week (1-2 cups serving size). You'll get all the benefits and keep your health on track. You may boil spinach for one minute in order to reduce the level of oxalates while maintaining the health benefits of this fantastic food.

When possible, choose fresh, organic spinach. Enjoy this leafy green as a salad, sautéed into a vegetable medley, layered in your lasagna, or boiled and added as a side dish to dinner. You'll reduce oxidative stress, prevent cancer, reduce inflammation, protect your heart, and boost your immune system; we can all appreciate these benefits.

Broccoli

This little green machine is packed with nutritional goodness! Broccoli comes from the Cabbage family and is closely related to cauliflower. Its color can range from dark green to a purple-green and its health benefits are worth a trip to the farmer's market or grocery store. Broccoli helps us detoxify, provides incredible antioxidant properties, helps us fight diseases like cancer and cardiovascular disease, all while reducing chronic inflammation in the body. You're going to want to make this a common food in your diet.

Here are the things you need to know about this green goddess:

Anti-inflammatory benefits:
- Broccoli helps reduce inflammation in the body.
- It contains Omega 3 fats which help lower the risk of an over active inflammatory system.
- Broccoli is full of isothiocyanates (ITC) which suppress the system that revs up our inflammatory response.

- Broccoli also helps reduce allergic and inflammatory reactions in the body by lowering IgE antibodies.

Antioxidant benefits:
- Broccoli has the most concentrated source of vitamin C.
- The phytonutrient content in broccoli helps promote and regulate the detoxification of our cells.
- The vitamin E content and minerals in broccoli lower the risk of oxidative stress in our body.

Cancer prevention:
- This beautiful food weakens the three pillars that cause cancer: oxidative stress, inadequate detoxification, and chronic inflammation.

Cardiovascular health benefits:
- Broccoli helps lower cholesterol and contains a load of B vitamins to provide cardiovascular benefits.
- The cardiovascular benefits of broccoli increase when steamed, but you do get a benefit eating it raw or cooked.

When you choose broccoli select one that is uniform in color and has a firm stalk. Store your broccoli in a plastic vegetable bag in the refrigerator. Let all the air out of the bag before storing. Only wash and cut the broccoli you're ready to eat; vitamin C content is lowered when broccoli is cut and stored.

We love broccoli in a yummy stir-fry, steamed and served with salmon and rice, added to our morning smoothie, or raw with humus. Dress it up any way you like and enjoy it daily.

Kale

Kale is my favorite go-to leafy green. There are multiple varieties to choose from; curly kale (this is what you most commonly see at the grocery store in bright green or purple color with large frilly-edged leaves), lacinato kale (also known as dinosaur kale, its leaf is long and narrow and more fibrous than the other varieties), and ornamental kale (this variety is a little more challenging to find and resembles a head of lettuce versus the bunch of leaves you find with the other varieties. The leaves are lighter in texture, often green, white or purple in color and are mildly flavored).

Our bones need both calcium and magnesium to be strong and flexible. One of the many beautiful qualities of kale is that is contains good amounts of both of these nutrients to support bone health. Magnesium is also necessary for many other important processes in the body so be sure to eat your kale to avoid the deficiency which many Americans suffer from.

Kale offers many of the same health benefits as other leafy greens: it provides cancer protection, protects the health of our eyes, offers the body excellent sources of vitamin C to protect our cells and reduce oxidative stress, and provides energy-producing vitamins and nutrients. One of the best benefits is that it's only 36 calories for one cup of kale. So enjoy this delicious food by adding it to smoothies, making a beautiful kale salad for lunch, or munching on kale chips.

Here's a favorite kale recipe of ours for you to enjoy.

RECIPE: *Crispy Kale Chips*

Ingredients

1 large bunch of leafy green kale

1 TBSP avocado oil

½ tsp garlic powder

½ tsp smoked paprika

⅛ tsp sea salt

⅛ tsp black pepper

Directions

- Preheat oven to 325°F.
- Wash kale thoroughly and remove leaves from the stem. Discard stem (or save to add to a smoothie). Lay the leaves of kale onto a clean kitchen towel. Place another towel over the layer of kale and roll like a burrito to gently dry the kale. Repeat this process until kale is completely dry.
- Break the leaves of kale into 3 inch by 3 inch pieces. Place the kale pieces into a large mixing bowl. Drizzle the avocado oil over the kale. Toss and massage the oil into the kale leaves so all the pieces are evenly coated. Add the spices, sea salt and pepper, tossing the kale to coat evenly.
- Line two baking sheets with parchment paper and create a single layer of kale chips on each baking sheet. Bake for 11-13 minutes or until the chips are crisp. Remove from the oven and allow the chips to cool. Serve as a snack or as a side to your favorite wrap or salad.

CHAPTER **19**

Eating Healthy with Smoothies, Tea…and Chocolate?

Sweet and savory come together in this chapter to provide additional ways to care for your cells. These foods might be less-obvious choices when it comes to eating healthy fare, but I guarantee you'll enjoy and appreciate them! Have fun creating new family recipes, adding these foods to your favorite snacks and meals, and feeling fabulous from the support they give your body.

Satiating Smoothies

It's important to balance your macronutrients when creating healthy smoothies for long-term satiation and balanced blood sugar. You'll pack a big punch of vitamins, minerals, fiber, and phytonutrients into your day when you create a healthy smoothie. Follow these tips to balance the goodness in your smoothie snack or meal.

Smoothie Tips:
Balance your macronutrients (protein, carbohydrates, fat).
- Helps stabilize sugar intake
- Provides quick and enduring energy
- Helps increase the metabolism

- Provides various nutrients and antioxidants to the body
- Helps with absorption of vitamins, minerals and nutrients

Balance fruit sugars with leafy greens and vegetables.

- Helps stabilize blood sugar
- Provides the body high amounts of various phytonutrients
- Helps fight disease with high antioxidant properties
- Provides good fiber for healthy digestion and removal of waste from the body
- Leafy greens are a great source of calcium and magnesium for strong bones and a healthy body

Use various fruits and vegetables for daily creations.

- Provides the body a variety of vitamins, minerals, and phyto-nutrients
- Food allergies and sensitivities are more prevalent when the same foods are consumed on a daily basis. Rotating your foods will help lower inflammation and ease sensitivities
- Each color in our food contains a variety of phytonutrients, which provide us our best disease-fighting properties. Eat a rainbow of color every day

Provide the body good sources of Omega 6 and Omega 3 fats.

- A ratio of 1:1 – 5:1 (Omega 6:Omega 3) is ideal for optimal health and to reduce inflammation in the body. Start with good fat in your smoothie and follow the guidelines for Omega 6 and Omega 3 in Chapter 17.

Select healthy protein sources.

- Stick with whole food sources as much as possible: organic and sprouted options are best
- Brown rice protein powder and hemp hearts are a favorite choice

- If protein powders aren't your thing, you can opt for whole sources of protein to accompany your breakfast smoothie: organic eggs, organic meats, quinoa hot cereal

Mix your greens first and then add berries and other fruit for a colorful smoothie.

RECIPE: *Morning Glory Smoothie*

Ingredients

1 cup coconut water

1 cup kale

½ of a large banana

½ cup frozen blueberries

3 frozen strawberries

5 chunks frozen pineapple

1 TBSP coconut oil

1 TBSP chia seeds

Directions

Blend the coconut water, kale and banana until smooth. Add frozen fruit, coconut oil and chia seeds and blend until smooth.

Variations: You may add a nut butter, hemp hearts, or brown rice protein powder for additional protein in your smoothie.

Green Tea

Green tea has a high concentration of phytonutrients, which, as you now know, lower our risk of disease, reduce free radicals, and even help us fight the common cold. Extensive research supports the many health benefits of green tea and let me tell you, it's time to get your 2-3 cups of it daily.

The health benefits of green tea extend from protective cardiovascular benefits to preventing osteoporosis.

- Green tea is known to reduce free radicals that often contribute to cardiovascular disease.
- Green tea offers cancer-preventative effects.
- Green tea can help stave off type 2 diabetes and may also improve glucose tolerance and insulin sensitivity in individuals with diabetes.
- Green tea supports healthy bones and teeth and aids in prevention of osteoporosis.

When purchasing green tea, look for loose-leaf options that produce a pale green to yellow-green cup of tea. This color is an indication that the tea is high quality. Place your tea bag in a cup, pour boiling water over the tea bag and let it steep for two to three minutes. Remove the tea bag from the cup and enjoy! You may also steep the tea in a larger glass container. Once you remove the tea bag you can cool the tea and serve over ice for iced green tea, one of my favorite treats on a hot summer day.

Raw Cacao: A Super Duper Food

Raw cacao (pronounced Ka-Cow) is a favorite of mine; how could it not be when it's the best form of chocolate you could provide your body?

The cacao beans come from the Theobroma cacao tree. While cocoa and cacao are two different words, they essentially mean the same thing although we generally use cocoa to refer to a more processed chocolate product with added sugar, versus the raw cacao, which has no sugar.

The forms of cacao you'll see most often are cacao nibs and cacao powder. Cacao nibs are cacao beans that have been roasted, separated from their husks, and broken into smaller pieces. Cacao powder is the nib ground into powder form and can be a wonderful addition to baked goods and smoothies.

Beyond the yummy, bitter chocolate taste of raw cacao come all the antioxidant and mineral benefits of the food. Note to all of you milk-chocolate lovers; it may take some time for you to get used to the flavor of cacao nibs and powder. Be patient and start by mixing it with other yumminess in your morning smoothie.

Cacao is known as the most potent antioxidant food in the world, which means it can serve our cells very well. When we have happy, healthy cells our body can thrive for a long time, and this is indeed why cacao is known as a "longevity" food. It helps people live well for a long time which is, I do believe, what all of us want.

The cacao bean is a great source of magnesium, which is needed for over 300 processes in our body. Among many things, magnesium is essential for muscle and nerve function and helps keep our heart in steady rhythm.

While you don't find fiber in a chocolate bar, raw cacao provides a hearty 9 grams of fiber in one ounce and has the highest amount of plant-based iron to keep our red blood cells happy. Raw cacao will help keep you alert as well with its all-natural stimulant effects.

A word of caution about raw cacao: cacao contains theobromine which is a nervous system stimulant and dilates blood vessels much like caffeine does. Start with small amounts of raw cacao, as some people are sensitive to this caffeine-like effect. You'll know best how to get the benefits from this amazing food while honoring your body's response. Start with small amounts and work up gradually.

Let's expand this chocolate conversation even more and dive into the benefits of dark chocolate.

Chocolate Chat

You just might agree with me when I say that happiness is even more plentiful when it includes a square of dark chocolate. While the magnificent flavor of dark chocolate ranks high in the list of reasons we enjoy the sweet treat, there's a long list of other reasons it should be a staple in our diet.

Dark chocolate is not to be mistaken with milk chocolate; the two are very different. Dark chocolate comes from the cacao bean, which is filled with phytonutrients. The cacao bean is roasted and used to create dark chocolate; raw dark chocolate refers to chocolate made with cacao beans that have not been roasted. This is where dark chocolate gets all of its health benefits, from the high amount of cacao found in the candy.

Cocoa powder is created when the roasted, husked and ground cacao bean is turned into a powder. During this process much of the fat is removed and you begin to lose nutrients. If you add milk and a bunch of sugar, you create milk chocolate. Milk chocolate should never be mistaken with dark chocolate because it is much higher in sugar and doesn't contain the same antioxidant and nutrient benefits as the dark chocolate. Do not be fooled into thinking all chocolate can serve you in health and happiness. You must select dark chocolate that is greater than 70% cacao or cocoa content.

The cacao content is what makes dark chocolate taste bitter, but it also provides the robust health benefits. It's a matter of finding the dark chocolate bar that provides you both the flavor and health benefits you desire. You might have to do a little taste testing to figure out which brand of bar you prefer most. One of my favorites is when sea salt is added to the dark chocolate; the flavor is outstanding and you increase your mineral content too!

There's a large amount of research to support the health benefits of dark chocolate. Dark chocolate not only feeds the body antioxidants, it is a known anti-inflammatory, and provides cardiovascular protection, reducing the risk of coronary heart disease, stroke, and diabetes. There are other benefits; dark chocolate has been shown to be anti-carcinogenic, helps lower the risk of Alzheimer's disease, and reduces symptoms of glaucoma and cataracts, to name a few.

The key to receiving the healthy benefits of dark chocolate is to be sure your dark chocolate contains 70% or greater cacao or cocoa content and to enjoy the chocolate in small amounts 2-3 times a day versus a large dose in one sitting.

As I always say, you gain the most health benefit from food that is closest to its whole form. If you appreciate the flavor of raw cacao you may add it to smoothies in the morning to give yourself a boost and soak up all the healthy benefits.

Your homework for the day is to feed your health and happiness with small amounts of dark chocolate. Enjoy!

Healthy Choices

Most often, when you ask people what they're doing to stay healthy, they'll comment that they exercise and eat well. I hope the last two chapters on caring for your cells has challenged you to think even more about the food selections you make, and how much these foods support your body. Your cells work hard to process, provide, heal and maintain the body so we can function at our best. Next time you take a bite of food, consider how its properties (phytonutrients, antioxidants, vitamins, and minerals) are serving you and give thanks for the amazing job they do!

We must consider the QUALITY of our food over QUANTITY. While the quantity of your food supports you in maintaining a healthy weight, it's the quality of your food that nourishes the cells of your body for long-term health.

CHAPTER 20

Healthy Family, Healthy You

"Why is there grass in the soup, mom?"

Tori couldn't understand at the age of five why there would be green grass in her soup, simply because it had never been there before. I explained that it wasn't grass, but rather spinach and it was in our soup because it helped make our bodies strong. I got lucky I guess because none of my crew has really questioned much of my cooking ever since. The kids were young when this healthy transition took place, but still needed to acquire new tastes and be open to trying new things.

Building a healthy family takes time and preparation. Getting everyone involved as much as possible will be in your favor, as we all tend to be more open to eating a new dish when we've had a hand in the making of it. Research suggests that we can retrain our taste buds with just 10-15 exposures to a food. This is one great reason to implement the "one bite rule" in your household. Over time, you'll all be more open to various foods and flavors just by the frequent exposure; I've seen this work with my own family. If need be, sneak yummy vegetables and leafy greens into meals in a stealthy manner by pureeing them and adding to sauces, soups and even baked goods. This stealth method works for young and adult children alike.

Involve the whole family as much as possible in your healthy transformation, discuss the reasons why you're making healthy change with one another, and share how proud you are of their openness to trying new things. You'll be amazed at how much kids can learn in a short period of time, and how good you and the family will feel as a result of your efforts.

This chapter is broken into a few sections to help you and the family with simple strategies for success. The first section focuses on raising healthy kids: it will be helpful for mentors, teachers, parents, and anyone who has children in their lives. Thereafter, the information is applicable for all; whether you're single or a family of ten. You'll be set with great lunch ideas for work and school, understand the health benefits of apple cider vinegar, and have natural cold and flu remedies at your fingertips (something we all contend with no matter our age).

Raising Healthy Kids

Once in a while, I have the wonderful pleasure of working with kids' groups; I teach them about nutrition and empower them to make good choices around food. We'll have discussions about the effects of eating bad food, and I often begin by asking them what might happen to their body if they eat junk food all the time. The only response I ever get is "it'll make me fat." And sometimes a sweet child will raise their hand and share how their parents already tell them they are too fat. These children are K-5th grade...

This breaks my heart for many reasons. I want to share these thoughts with you around the health of our children. Below are seven easy steps to follow that will groom the little loves in your life to cherish their body, listen to the needs of their body, and feel great about the decisions they make for themselves.

Kids eat what they're provided: Do not expect your child to have willpower when it comes to candy, bagels, cereal, chips, and cookies! The adult in charge of the grocery shopping brings food into the home to feed the family. If your goal is to create health for your family, you need to clean out the pantry and fridge and only restock with those foods that align with your goals. As a parent, I went through a feeling of guilt when I drastically changed our diet. I felt bad that my kids no longer had packaged fruit chews and chocolate chip cookies around for their pleasure every day. Here's what I've learned: kids might put up a fuss in the beginning, but they move on, they appreciate the structure and goodness of the food you serve them, and feel amazing for it. Kick guilt to the curb and start providing what you believe is best for your family.

Behavior make-over: Sugar, food coloring, preservatives, hydrogenated fat and more fill the boxes of processed foods. All of these ingredients harm our children in one fashion or another—sugar addiction, ADHD, cancer, heart disease, and more. Sugar wreaks havoc on their ability to focus, their energy level will be fluctuating all day, they'll experience headaches and irritability, and make unhealthy choices. It takes years for disease to set in. These little guys and gals are still growing and developing; it's incredibly important they have every bit of nourishment to do just that in the healthiest manner possible.

Thin doesn't mean healthy. So many kiddos equate being "fat" to being unhealthy. I love sharing with them that I've been an athlete my whole life, fit and thin, but I still got very, very sick because I ate a lot of the wrong kinds of food. Start having conversations with your kids about the need to give our body/organs the right "fuel" to keep everything running in tip-top shape. Use the example of a car: you buy the most expensive dream car (think big here) and instead of putting the highest grade fuel in the tank, you select the cheapest stuff. You forget to give it an oil change every few months, you never rotate the tires or get a full tune-up. Even though you might be washing your car every day and it's looking beautiful on the outside, things start going wrong. It doesn't gather speed as efficiently, it starts sputtering, warning lights appear on the dashboard, and your smooth ride feels bumpy because things aren't balanced. Eventually, your beautiful car breaks down on the side of the road. Our bodies are no different. We need to be a well-oiled machine, getting a good tune up here and there, selecting the right fuel, and running efficiently. While it is difficult for a body to carry extra weight, being "fat" is not the only indicator of disease.

Teach them to listen to their body. Kids are keen, and in tune with their surroundings. Have they experienced a sniffle today? Maybe they're tired, have a headache, can't focus, or are feeling irritable. Food largely impacts performance in the classroom and on the sports field. Investigate how they're feeling with their diet, sleep patterns, and stress. Make adjustments and note the positive changes.

Life is going to happen. There are times of celebration and events that might offer us lower-quality food options. Children should understand that there are "sometimes foods" and "always foods" to choose from. "Always foods" include our plant-based foods that come from the earth as well as high-quality organic animal foods. "Sometimes foods" are those that are prepackaged, or high in sugar even when baked from scratch. There should be no guilt associated with food, but rather an empowering, free feeling to make the choices that best serve you. Celebrate when it's time and do your best to fill in all the other times with "always foods."

Notice how your body feels in each circumstance and learn from your experience. When you and your children live this way, you'll have a healthy relationship with food. No restriction, no calorie counting. Do your best and feel good about it.

Help them glow. Children want to do well, learn, and have a choice in every matter. They are wise beyond their years; my kids could read a complicated food label and tell me whether it's good for us or not at the young age of seven. Include children in the process, celebrate the incredible beings they are, and always encourage them to take an active role in their health. Ask them what they love most about themselves. I think you'll be surprised when some don't have an answer. In time they should list off a dozen things to celebrate and love about themselves and it is my hope that not one thing has to do with the way they look.

Take charge of the menu. Most restaurants have children's menu items that include hot dogs, mac-n-cheese, pizza, spaghetti, or a hamburger. Often, there's not one veggie on the plate unless it's in the form of a French fry. Let your kids order off the adult menu, share an entrée with them or have multiple kids share one. It's worth the little extra money and their long-term health.

Lunch Box Tidbits (for Adults Too)

Lunch tends to be one of those last-minute, throw-together meals for the whole family and when it comes to packing the lunch box there tends to be very little variety. I've frequented school lunch rooms and have felt very sad looking at all the lunch boxes filled with prepackaged goods: Lunchables, pudding, cheese-n-cracker snacks, premade PB&J frozen sandwiches, and chips. I rarely see a box full of fresh fruit and vegetables, or a healthy entrée for the child to eat. Unfortunately, this same theme tends to find its way into the workplace but instead of Lunchables, folks are throwing prepackaged meals into the microwave, or depending on 100 calorie packs and PB&J to suffice.

I realize that we're all busy and our household is no different; balancing work, school, kid's activities, groceries, cleaning, cooking, and more. The fact is that if you do a little prep work on the weekend, cleaning all your vegetables, preparing entrées and a pot of soup to be used during the week, and mapping out what the lunch menu looks like for everyone, you can have everyone's lunchboxes filled with nutritious food in 15 minutes or less every day. It doesn't need to be fancy, or over the top, just nutritious so you all have the support you need for a healthy, focused, and energetic day.

Involve the whole family when creating a meal plan for the week of lunches, and have everyone help with prepping and packing lunches. It takes less time when everyone pitches in and when the kids are involved they take pride in their work and are more apt to eat what they're being provided. Here are some tips and ideas for easy, nutritious lunches.

The Thermos

It's a homemade meal's best friend and makes life easy for the person making the lunches.

Double your dinner recipe so you have an extra serving for all family members to enjoy for lunch the next day.

Soups, spaghetti, beans and rice, quinoa, veggies and chicken, and chili are easy things to pack up for lunch.

The key is to heat your thermos before filling it up with food. Pour boiling water into the thermos, cover, and let sit for 10 minutes while you're warming up the meal on the stove. When 10 minutes has passed, dump the water out and dish your hot food into the thermos for warm-keeping until the lunch break begins.

Variety

We can all get easily bored with the same food day in and day out. Spice things up a bit in easy, healthy ways.

Pack a variety of veggies and fruit every day. You can mix things up by creating fruit salads, serving organic unsweetened applesauce, using a fancy slicer to cut your cucumbers and carrots, and make it fun by creating colorful patterns in the dish or on a skewer (just no sharp ends for the kids, please).

Serve a variety of raw, roasted, steamed, and sautéed vegetables and play around with various seasonings: cumin, turmeric, rosemary, garlic, thyme, salt and pepper.

Provide various dips to enjoy with your veggies. Hummus, bean dip, even Ranch will do the trick. If it helps you get good phytonutrients, vitamins and minerals into your body, then pack the dip and let everyone enjoy!

Kids, and adults alike, tend to have minimal time to enjoy their lunch so make things as easy as possible for everyone. Peel the orange, slice the apple, and dice the peppers.

Drinks

We all know the consequences of filling up on sugar in the middle of the day. Productivity and energy go down, and we're ready for a nap. Set your kids up for best success!

Water is essential for every process in our body, and most people don't get enough of it. Grab a fun water bottle to include in your child's lunchbox and provide water for them to drink at lunch. Make sure you have a glass or stainless steel water bottle to drink from all day long at your desk or in the car if you're traveling. It'll save you from spending on packaged drinks that are usually full of sugar, corn syrup, food coloring and added flavors. This is not what we want anyone to fuel up for a productive day.

You can spruce up your water by adding lemon, strawberry, cucumber or even mint. Let the kids be adventurous over the weekend with adding fruit and veggies to the water to see what they like.

Protein, Carbs and Fat

Our kids (and us too) need to be creative, on-task, and energetic. This means we need to have a balance of protein, carbohydrates, and fat in our lunch box every day.

- Use avocado as a spread on wraps and sandwiches.
- Cook with olive oil, avocado oil, or coconut oil for meal making and thermos lunches.
- Provide a nut and fruit trail mix as a snack.
- Include nitrite/nitrate free deli meats, cheese, chicken, turkey, beans, and eggs in the lunch for good sources of protein.
- Pack a nutritious punch with lots of veggies and fruit!
- Whole grains keep you fuller for longer: think brown rice, quinoa, oats, and barley.

I'm here to support you through your health journey; visit my website for additional recipes and resources.

Apple Cider Vinegar: A Pantry Staple

Apple Cider Vinegar (ACV) is a must-have for healthy living. It can be used for the health of our body, and our home and our pets can benefit from it too. The key to receiving the health benefits of ACV are to purchase an organic, raw, unfiltered and unprocessed option. Bragg brand is my favorite. In case you're wondering, the little floaties in the bottle are normal and we need them. They are the live probiotic portion of the vinegar and a sign of a high-quality product. The floaties are responsible for the health benefits we receive from the ACV.

Let's talk health benefits. Here are 15 reasons you want to make this a pantry staple and start using it today:

1. ACV can help alkalize the body when accompanied by a plant-based diet. An alkaline environment helps inhibit the growth of fungus, bacteria, and parasites which means you'll be better able to fight off the common cold and flu.

2. Got a sore throat? ACV is believed to have anti-bacterial properties that can help soothe your throat in quick fashion. Gargle with ACV in order to relieve pain and expedite your recovery.

3. ACV is an all-natural, cost-effective teeth whitener. Rub the teeth directly with ACV and rinse with water.

4. Sip on it for an energy boost! One of my favorite ways to consume ACV is to add 2 tablespoons to 10 ounces of boiling water. Add a teaspoon of local honey or agave nectar and sip on it like tea. You'll receive all the health benefits as well as a boost of energy.

5. Research suggests that ACV can help relieve heartburn by correcting low acid levels. Experts state you should feel relief in short order after taking a teaspoon of ACV followed by a glass of water.

6. ACV will boost your hair's body and shine. Mix ½ tablespoon with a cup of cold water and use it as a rinse after shampooing (may be used several times a week for dramatic results). It can also help get rid of a flaky scalp.

7. ACV can help your body detox and stimulate cardiovascular circulation. Because of its alkalizing effects, it breaks up mucous in the body, helps detoxify the liver, and creates an overall detoxification of the body.

8. Fatigue, brain fog, sugar cravings and yeast infections are usually associated with too much candida in your system. ACV is rich in natural enzymes that can help rid your body of candida and

get you back to balanced health. Be sure to avoid sugar while you're getting rid of candida, or you'll be counteracting all your effort.

9. Data shows that you can achieve weight loss benefits from sustained daily intake of acetic acid (which happens to be a main ingredient in ACV). One study found that subjects that consumed acetic acid for 12 weeks experienced significant declines in body weight, abdominal fat, waist circumference and triglycerides. For daily weight management, add 2 teaspoons of ACV to 16 ounces of water.

10. Home is in need of a detox too. We often use too many chemical cleaners that can be toxic to our system when we have natural alternatives to use. ACV is one of these easy alternatives you can use to freshen up the home. It can be mixed with water and used to clean the bathroom, kitchen, countertops, and the floors. If you'd like an all-natural fabric softener you may add ½ cup of ACV to your wash and condition your clothes.

11. Give your furry friend a hand. Get rid of fleas by diluting the ACV by 50% water and use a spray bottle to spray the mixture onto your pet's fur. Rub it in and let dry.

12. Bug bite aid: soak a cotton ball in ACV and dab it on bug bites and other minor skin irritations to relieve pain and swelling.

13. Use ACV as an acid for salad dressings, soups, and stews. It will add wonderful flavor. If you add too much, you can always counterbalance the taste with a bit of Grade B Maple Syrup.

14. Get moving: ACV can help loosen the bowels. Take a shot or two when feeling a little backed up and it'll help flush out your system.

15. ACV is known to help reduce pain and inflammation associated with arthritis.

While it may take some getting used to, introducing apple cider vinegar into your life is well worth it. Know that it will help you regain and maintain good health so you may enjoy life to the fullest!

Natural Remedies for Cold and Flu

We receive many blessings through the winter and holiday months, but a cold and flu we can do without. Take a proactive approach to protect your body and when you do experience the symptoms of a cold and flu, use these natural remedies to heal up quickly.

Be proactive by doing the following:

- Avoid "white foods": bagels, bread, pasta, white rice, cookies, muffins, etc.
- Avoid sugary sweets: candy, cookies, cakes, ice cream, cinnamon rolls.
- Drink two cups of green tea daily.
- Get ample rest: a minimum of 7-8 hours a night is ideal for adults, children need 10-11.
- Boost your vitamin C: eat leafy greens, broccoli, peppers, berries, and oranges.
- Take Epsom salt baths: soak for 20 min in a hot Epsom salt bath to detoxify the body.
- Eat plenty of onions and garlic: chop each and let set for 5-10 min before cooking to enhance the antibacterial/antiviral properties of each.
- Eat lots of plant-based foods: leafy greens, vegetables, fruit, whole grains, beans, nuts and seeds.

When a cold or flu does strike, follow all the proactive tips and add these into your arsenal:

Garlic: For a sore throat, peel the garlic clove and keep it whole. Place the whole clove in your cheek and suck on it for 10 minutes.

If you experience any burning please remove the clove as burning is not healthy or necessary. Garlic has antibacterial and antifungal properties and can aid to fight off many illnesses. It'll stop your sore throat in its tracks.

Ingesting garlic is very beneficial. Peel the garlic clove, and mince. Let it set out in the room air for five minutes to enhance its antibacterial properties. Place chopped garlic in a small glass of water and drink it quickly, without chewing. For children, it is best to mince the garlic and put it in a bite of applesauce. Have your child take a bite of applesauce and immediately swallow it without chewing.

Cinnamon is another natural antibacterial and antiviral. Mix one tablespoon of cinnamon with a teaspoon of honey, add boiling water to make a hot tea. It'll help alleviate a sore throat and congestion and may aid in reducing fever.

Apple cider vinegar: add one tablespoon of Braggs brand ACV to water (I prefer boiling water) and add one teaspoon of agave nectar and enjoy. This drink will help alkalize the gut, which will help kill off bacteria and viruses.

Zinc can help respiratory symptoms and minimize the reproduction of cold and flu viruses. You may take zinc in a lozenge or supplement form. Please follow dosing recommendations on the packaging.

Peppermint oil can be used to aid in digestion and to lower fever. It is antimicrobial and antiviral. Use it as a tea or rub the oil on the feet of the ill person to help reduce fever.

Oregano oil: This is a personal favorite of mine. Oregano oil is a potent antibiotic and antiviral. For a sore throat, dilute 4-5 drops of oregano oil in water and use as a gargle and spit it out. DO NOT ingest oregano oil. While the taste is less than desirable, the effects are robust. Your sore throat will feel relief! You may also use oregano oil on the feet of the ill person to aid in killing off bacteria and viruses.

Hydrate: The body is in need of extra fluids anytime you're feeling ill. Hot fluids like herbal tea, green tea or the honey/cinnamon or apple cider vinegar drinks I mentioned are great, but be sure to give the body plenty of fresh water as well.

The body is going to experience illness at times; it's not a bad thing. Do your best to stay well by nourishing the body with good nutrients, getting ample rest, exercising, and making choices that serve you well. When illness does strike, follow the tips I have provided you and give your body extra TLC.

In order to keep your family healthy all year long, focus on the food first and implement the natural remedies when needed. Food is the foundation of health. Fill up on bright, colorful whole foods and do your best to avoid the prepackaged foods and products that are going to negate your health.

This concludes our section on the power of food, and building a healthy foundation. Be sure to go back and reference it when you have questions, need support, or want to try something new. There's plenty of information to work with!

The last section you're headed into is all about nurturing yourself through the journey. Everything you've learned so far will nourish the body for long-term health; the information, stories and insights in the pages to come will help you honor your healthy boundaries, encourage you to savor every moment, and create a new normal for yourself. Get your pen ready, there's more work to be done!

SECTION III

The Care and Keeping of You

The Dalai Lama, when asked what surprised him most about humanity, answered, "Man. Because he sacrifices his health in order to make money. Then he sacrifices money to recuperate his health. And then he is so anxious about the future that he does not enjoy the present; the result being that he does not live in the present or the future; he lives as if he is never going to die, and then dies having never really lived."

This quote found me a few years ago and has stuck with me ever since. Maybe it'll make you pause, just as it did for me. After reading it I really stopped to consider how I wanted live for the rest of my days and reflect on how I was caring for my body. The beautiful thing about having a choice in how we live is that we can always decide to choose differently when life isn't what we want it to be. This last section focuses on self-care so you may continue to build on your health each and every day. You'll be challenged to release the unnecessary, and learn to savor the small moments. Enjoy all of it. Have fun strengthening your foundation, and be proud of the work you're doing to care for the one-and-only brilliant YOU!

CHAPTER 21

Choice

It is my firm belief that optimal health can only be achieved when you balance your table food and life food. If you remember from the beginning of the book, table food is all the food we put in our body to provide nourishment. Life food is everything outside of the food we consume that impacts our health. We'll be focused on life food in this section; it's all about nurturing yourself and making sure that you're caring for yourself in the best manner as you continue on your journey to healthy, vibrant living.

I loved listening to the thought leaders on stage at Oprah's The Life You Want Tour. A beautiful friend had gifted me a ticket, and we were graced with the presence of Oprah, Elizabeth Gilbert, Mark Nepo, Rob Bell and Iyanla Vanzant. I scribbled many notes in those hours as their words burrowed into my heart and mind. It was an experience of shift, grace, inspiration, and possibility.

At this point in my career, I was comfortably living with my body, my health, and my life, and inspiring others to do the same through speaking and coaching. But Rob Bell said something that made me pause for one looooong moment; he changed the way I look at things with four simple words. While I believe I have a pretty positive outlook on most things in life, the day to day mundane tasks are not always something I greet with true excitement or pleasure. I will often get wrapped up in the need to do them, and sometimes even get frustrated feeling that nobody else in my household is helping me out.

I've used these four words every day since hearing Rob speak, and it's changed my outlook, shifted perspective in all areas of life, and has provided me increased joy and happiness. I am quite confident they'll do the same for you! The four words are "Wow, I get to…" They sound simple, but are truly powerful. I can't wait to share more about this powerful gift of words later in this chapter!

How would life improve for you if there were no "have to's" and you were able to say no without explanation anytime you needed to do so? If someone had asked this of me five years ago I probably would have sarcastically laughed because I never would have thought it possible to achieve. Most of us are givers, lovers and pleasers; myself included! The deal is we can be all these things and more if that's what we desire. But we must find ways to do so that feed our health, bring joy to our lives, and align with the healthy boundaries and life rules we've created for ourselves. Let's begin with the "have to" syndrome; it's a great launching pad into this topic.

The "Have To" Syndrome

You and only you are responsible for every choice you make. There's no need to blame your job, your family, a broken relationship, or the weather. Everything you do is based on the choices you make; but not everyone always sees it this way and that leads me to the "have to" syndrome.

The "have to" syndrome is my not-so-scientific diagnosis to describe the people who make choices because they feel they "have to" because of an expectation or need, even when that choice contradicts what they really desire to do for their own happiness and joy. While I see this occur every day, it is exacerbated during the holidays when expectations and stress are high, and responsibilities are great. Can you hear your own "have to's" running through your mind? "I have to send out Christmas cards." "I have to travel to see family when all I really want to do is hang out at home." "I have to find the perfect gift."

We create our own happiness through our choices. When we make intentional choices, we can focus on the reason for our decision and in turn experience more joy. Let's take, for instance, the example of having to travel to see family for the holidays, when all you really want to do is relax in your own home and start creating your own traditions.

If you've always traveled to see family, there's probably an expectation that you'll continue to do so every year. Your family will be incredibly happy to see you and you'll be happy to see them too. But while you make the decision, all you can think about is how you HAVE to go see everyone, because you've always done so and people will be greatly disappointed if you were to choose differently. You can't bear to think of the disappointment, the guilt you will feel, or the complaints you may hear as a result. So you go, all the while wishing that you had stood up for yourself, and stayed home as you wished. In this scenario, you may very well end up enjoying yourself, but your decision was made because you felt like you had to, versus making the intentional decision from a place of happiness. This isn't to say you should never go see your family for the holidays; but if you choose to do so, that choice needs to come from your place of gratitude, love, happiness, and joy. The only "have to's" that exist in this life are those that you put on yourself.

When you work from a place of gratitude, things will flow easily, you'll experience happiness and joy, and feel fulfilled. Back to our example: if you were to contemplate your reasons, you may discover that even though you'd like to stay home, you do value the family time together; you enjoy mom's homemade holiday treats, the interaction with your siblings, and the opportunity for your children to create life long memories with their cousins. If you were to decide to travel to the family as a result of these things, you could focus on all the joy you'll experience by making the trip. On the other hand, you might realize that it's too much work to travel, everyone is tired, and while you'd love to see the family you really desire to wake up in your own home on Christmas morning and make your own holiday treats. You decide you aren't going this year, because you know that you'll experience greater joy and relaxation in your own home. You'll feel empowered by your decision, and even though there may be disappointment as a result, you'll know that you made the right choice for you. This choice will feed the opportunity for you to make even more intentional choices in your life which will result in increased peace and joy.

There are two other things to consider when making an intentional choice:

1. You are not responsible for others' reactions or another person's journey.
2. Your mindset can make all the difference in the world.

Allow people the freedom to react as they need to react. Release the need to control the situation and know that they're on their own life journey and you are on yours. People don't always love the fact that you make choices that serve you well, that you feel happiness and joy, and are empowered to do well for yourself. If you experience any of these things, please stay true to yourself; breathe deeply and on the out-breath release the need to control the situation. Know that you're serving yourself in the healthiest, happiest manner possible. You create your own happiness through the choices you make.

If you find yourself in a negative place, or in that complaining mode about having to do something, please do this one thing. Trade the words "I have to do this" with "Wow, I get to do this," and say it with the enthusiasm of a small child experiencing a merry-go-round for the first time. Feel the joy, the gratitude, the excitement for the opportunity to be able to do such a task, or activity. You can use this when you head over to the sink of dirty dishes, when you care for a sick child all night, or when you have to work late three nights in a row to meet a project deadline. One should feel so blessed to be able to have dirty dishes to wash because it means you had food to eat, or care for a sick child because even though you're exhausted you should be so blessed to be the one there for them, or to work late on a project because you should be so blessed to have a stable job that allows you to live the life you desire. There are small gifts everywhere and many reasons to give thanks and express gratitude. Choose this mindset, choose happiness, and believe that you deserve every bit of it.

The only "have to's" that exist in life are those that you put on yourself. Make intentional choices that come from a place of gratitude and ask yourself how it'll serve you to make one decision over another. When you're happy and healthy, you'll better serve others and in turn they'll begin experiencing more happiness, too.

What is one "have to" you can release yourself of today? It can be in your home life or work life.

✕ EXERCISE: *My "Have To's"*

What "have to's" exist in your life?

_____

_____

_____

_____

_____

_____

What steps will you take to release the "have to" syndrome and move forward in a healthy manner?

_____

_____

_____

_____

_____

_____

_____

Have to's exist everywhere in our lives. Think of how many work meetings involve some type of food, how many cakes are made to celebrate birthdays and graduations, or how many people fill up on Velveeta cheese product dips on Super Bowl Sunday! I'm not saying you have to ditch all of this (well, maybe the Velveeta cheese) but you can do what you want to do; the only have to's are those you allow in your life. Meet colleagues for a walking meeting, serve fresh berries and fresh whipped cream for the birthday, and if you're going to make nacho dip for the game at least start with whole-food organic cheese. It's about making healthy choices in every area of our life.

No is a Complete Sentence

No. It's a one-word complete sentence, but have you ever felt the need to say more? So often an explanation will follow this powerful word, but why? I'll be the first to admit that I had a difficult time ever saying "no" to anyone or anything; and if I did say "no" I always followed it up with a good explanation.

In the "yes" days, my husband had a line he threw at me all the time: "You don't have to be the hero." This incredible man of mine saw my "need to please" long before I recognized it. The "hero line" came up when I stayed up 'til midnight baking cupcakes for the bake sale, took the lead and organized the school's fall festival, or made a three-hour gourmet dinner for friends when quick lasagna would do the trick. It took a long time before simple started to trump heroism.

When I look back, it wasn't the act of giving that caused my husband to call me out, but rather that he saw me suffering as a result of my choices, especially in the days of illness. Giving to others is a beautiful gift. The only problem is that if you give beyond your means, you end up in a deficit. I'm not talking financial means, although the same rule would apply; I'm talking about your physical, emotional, and healthy means. What good can you give to others if there's no good left to give to yourself? This is the question to ask when making decisions about the activities and responsibilities in your life. There will always be an expectation, there will always be someone needing help. While we cannot be all to everyone, we can selectively choose to give, in the best way we know how, for the best period of time, that serves ourselves and our family, in the healthiest manner.

Practice makes perfect. Start saying "No" when it best serves you to do so. It can be said in a kind, loving manner or forcefully if necessary. You can share that you'd like to serve another time when life allows, if you desire, but there's no need for explanation. No. It's enough, a one-word, complete sentence.

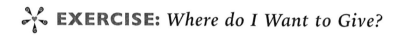 EXERCISE: *Where do I Want to Give?*

List three areas of your life that you'd like to donate time, energy, or money to this year:

1._____
2._____
3._____

Now, you'll need to stick to your list, honor your emotional, physical, and family needs and say no when necessary. I know, it's easier said than done. Have every confidence in yourself and own your power! We can't possibly give everything to everyone, and when we're selective about where, when, and how we'd like to donate our time and effort, we can focus and do a great job while taking care of ourselves along the way.

Start exercising your right to say "No" in a kind and beautiful way that supports you, your health, and life goals. Each experience will build on the next, and soon you'll be following your healthy boundaries with ease just by using the simple word "no"... followed by a thank you.

Using Your Voice

I'm not talking about singing in the shower every morning...although that is something I enjoy every day! Using your voice means speaking up, sharing your thoughts, providing direction, and openly communicating your needs. We are all conditioned to respond in certain ways. I learned at a young age not to rock the boat; it was better to keep the peace than to speak up and use my voice. The hard part is that while this may have served me well in my younger years, it certainly didn't in my adulthood.

What do you need to let go of in order to use your voice? Keeping the peace in my adult years meant not sharing my feelings with others—my husband, my siblings, my parents, my friends. I would do whatever I needed to do to keep the peace and people please, and it caused me more stress than necessary. I always questioned myself and my decisions, and this response mechanism certainly contributed to my ill body. I was the adult but that 10-year old girl who wanted to keep quiet, avoid conflict, and make sure nobody was upset was shining through all the time. Something needed to change for me to create healthier, happier relationships. I had to be able to say what I needed to say without feeling like the world would fall apart if I did so.

A big turning point took place for me early on in my dating years with my husband. I was upset, and as always, I clammed up, got quiet and didn't want to speak about it. He sat me on the couch and told me that I needed to share what was bothering me, and that he couldn't do anything to help the situation until I did so. It didn't work. So we sat there, and sat there, and he finally said, "I'll sit here all day; we aren't getting off the couch until you tell me what is wrong." It wasn't that I was afraid of speaking; I was afraid that if I shared what was wrong, he might walk away as a result. This was part of my conditioning. Our subconscious thoughts do not judge or assess a situation to figure out whether our reaction is healthy or applicable.

We sat there for a while longer and in the end I did speak up. And guess what? He didn't walk away, and I felt like the world had been lifted off my shoulders. Through the years I've continued to work on this, albeit it's a difficult task at times. Now that we're 15 years into marriage I'm sure there are days he'd probably appreciate that quiet person who never rocked the boat, but at least he always knows where I stand.

❊ EXERCISE: *My Voice*

While it may be challenging, because you're breaking a cycle you've known all your life, it's empowering to express your feelings and use your voice. Practice doing this today. Think of a situation where you really wished you could've shared your thoughts, but held back due to fear around how the person may have reacted. What would you have said? How would you have felt being able to use your voice? What will it provide you to do so in the future?

What would you have said?

_____

_____

_____

_____

_____

_____

How would you have felt being able to use your voice?

_____

_____

What will it provide you to do so in the future?

This is a big step; take a minute to read over your entry. You were given a beautiful, strong voice to be used to communicate with others in your life. You may do so with grace, love and kindness always, but the big thing here is that you must do so. No more staying small, no more keeping the peace for the sake of others, and no more worrying about what others may think if you stand up for yourself and speak your truth. Begin using your voice and notice how your life opens up as you do.

CHAPTER 22

Be Vulnerable, Savor, and Enjoy

This chapter is full of savory treats that'll help you slow down, tap into the life events and activities that bring you most joy, and get a good laugh! Exploring fulfillment can cause vulnerability and begs for reflection on your life. Enjoy the exercises and feel free to bare it all; you'll make remarkable strides!

A friend of mine was visiting and we got into a conversation about the book that I was writing (which happens to be the one you're holding right now). She said, "You must be so excited to have it almost finished." While I did feel excited, I told her that I also felt very vulnerable. I remember feeling this way when I opened my coaching practice, and the first time I stood on stage to speak to a large group; there are so many "ifs" that run through the mind. The thing is, when we can step through the fear, and embrace the vulnerability, we feel fulfilled and are able to spread our wings and fly.

Baring It All

Before catching a flight back home one day, I decided to connect with nature on an hour-long walk. The air was crisp, and the sunshine lit up the blue California sky. I'm always inspired by nature, but that day everything seemed raw and stripped down. Pine needles covered the ground and the trees were losing many of their red, orange and yellow leaves. Little squirrels played chase around the trunks of the ponderosa pines while others collected acorns from the ground; I thought of all the work they'd need to do to prepare for winter to arrive.

There's something genuinely beautiful about the trees baring themselves; losing their leaves and needles, they show off their many knots, scars, and weathered beauty. It's a season in their life cycle that allows them to shed what is no longer necessary, and as a result, allows new life in.

What if you were to bare all just as the trees do in the fall and shed what is no longer necessary? We function differently than the tree; we have a choice, and we also experience fear and vulnerability. The question still begs to be asked; what if you were to shed what is no longer necessary?

When we step through our fear and open ourselves to vulnerability, we're able to be fulfilled. Just as with the tree, it is time for you to shed what is no longer necessary in order to let new life in.

In the coming week I'd like you to keep this page near you throughout the day. Be very aware of your daily routine, your relationships, and habits. How are these things in your life serving you in a positive way? What things could you release so new life can be welcomed in?

Keep a running list of things as they come to you. Maybe it's time to purge the pantry, donate the clothes that no longer serve you, or have a heart to heart conversation with a loved one. While the need for release is a common thread for all, the list you create will be unique for you.

There's so much we can learn about ourselves when we decide to follow nature's guidance. In times of chaos we can tap into the stillness of the tree. When you feel the need to control everything, you can observe how water flows right over the boulders and rocks that sit in its way. We all need different things at different times in our lives. What element in nature do you need to connect with most right now?

Take time to observe your environment, relationships, activities, and responsibilities. Journal about the things in life that are positively serving you as well as those things that may need to be released in order for you to achieve health and happiness.

❖ EXERCISE: *Joy and Release*

These things serve me in a positive way:

1._____
2._____
3._____
4._____
5._____
6._____
7._____
8._____
9._____
10._____

These things could be released so I may welcome new life in:

1._____
2._____
3._____
4._____

5._____

6._____

7._____

8._____

9._____

10._____

What part of nature do you need to connect most with right now?

_____

_____

_____

_____

_____

_____

The Yumminess in Life

Are you fulfilled, or just feeling full? Food may fill you up, but it doesn't provide you fulfillment. It's the yumminess in life that allows us to feel joy and happiness.

Travel back to your childhood…what did you love to do most? I remember the summer days where my younger siblings and I would play outside all day, in the sandbox, spraying the hose at each other, making mud pies and soaking up the sun. When mom called us in for dinner, we would gripe and want nothing to do with it…because we were completely fulfilled, in our space of happiness and sun. We didn't need any other food to feed us.

As we age, our life food suffers a bit. We have more responsibilities than we did in our younger years and most often those good ol' summer days in the sandbox fall way to the bottom of the to-do list. We find ourselves filling these voids with table food, and most often it's not the nourishing food our body needs, as we feed cravings for sugar or salty treats.

What is it that you loved to do in your childhood? If it was painting, then get your easel out and start a new paint project. Maybe you enjoyed hiking with the family; set a day and time to hike with your family or friends, or maybe just enjoy this time for yourself. I may not head back to the sandbox in my 40s but a nice beach vacation, or connection with friends and family for a day in the sun, would provide me the same fulfilling experience. Take charge and create an opportunity for fulfillment—no more just feeling full.

EXERCISE: *Fulfillment*

What activities/hobbies/events did you love as a child?

_____

_____

_____

_____

_____

_____

How could you incorporate these activities/hobbies/events into your life today?

_____

_____

_____

_____

_____

_____

Learn to Savor

We may occasionally think about savoring a bite of food, or savoring a special moment, but today I'd like to talk about savoring some "normal" moments in your day. Take time out for you: to breathe, be present, and find beauty in the simple things.

Summer vacations offer great opportunity to step away from the normal grind, unplug the phone and computer, and relish in what is. I find it hard not to do so when my toes are deep in the sand, the sun shines brightly on my face and the light breeze whisks through my hair. The repetitive sound of the rolling waves causes my mind to explore all that is possible, and provides peace to my day. I'm sure you've had moments like this. If only we could transport ourselves to this beautiful place when we're back to our work, when the pressure is on, our schedule is tight, and we feel like there are too few hours in the day to accomplish all we need to do.

The simple fact of the matter is we can get to this peaceful place, and allow our mind to explore all that is possible even in the midst of chaos or a stressful time. It just takes a little focus and dedication.

Practice these simple steps and start savoring the "normal" moments in your day:

1. Begin each day with gratitude. State five things you're grateful for before getting out of bed to start your day.
2. Focus on one thing at a time; be present with the one task you're working on, or with the one person you're with.
3. Function with a "can do" attitude. All things are possible; there are many ways to solve a problem. Figure out what works best for you and the situation and move forward with a plan.
4. Breathe. Take nice deep breaths, the ones that fill your whole belly! Then exhale all the air out of your belly and repeat the cycle. Do this every hour for one minute and you'll experience more calm in your day.

5. Think about what is important to you in this life (family, relationships, good work ethic, exercise, healthy eating, and whatever else speaks to you). Prioritize these things and be present with the important people and activities in your life. When you are truly present, and focused on that one beautiful thing that is important to you, you'll experience what it feels like to savor a "normal" moment.

6. End the day with gratitude: Before falling into restful sleep, write down 10 things that you're grateful for in your gratitude journal. Focus on the simple moments in your day; the smile you received from a stranger, the beautiful colors in the garden or the simple fact that you were able to problem solve and move forward with a solution.

None of this takes a great amount of time or effort, but rather a few minutes of time consistently throughout your day. It is with this consistent dedication and implementation that you'll begin to feel the calm, and savor the simple or "normal" moments in life, just as you do the big ones.

Laugh Every Day

"Sometimes crying or laughing are the only options left, and laughing feels better right now." ~ Veronica Roth, Divergent

Here's My Contribution to Healthy Laughter Today...

It had been one of those days of running from one thing to the next. Before I realized it, it was 9:30 p.m. and I still had to run to the grocery store. I must not have hydrated well, because my lips were feeling pretty chapped and dry. On the short drive, I reached into my purse in the dark of the car and pulled out what I thought was my minty Burt's Bees lip balm. I took full advantage of this moistening opportunity, running the lip balm in a circular motion around my lips and surrounding skin. Pure relief!

While grabbing my groceries I said hello to a few employees. It seemed that people were a bit subdued; maybe it was because it was so late. I remember thinking the people I encountered were acting a bit "off."

After the 45-minute shopping trip (which was only supposed to be a 15 minute quick run), I returned home. While I was carrying bags into the house, my husband looked at me and said, "Oh my gosh babe, what's wrong with your mouth?"

"What?" I said.

He said, "Something is wrong with your lips; I think you might be having an allergic reaction, look in the mirror!" I rushed over to the mirror and took a peek at my ailing mouth...and then busted out laughing in embarrassment and amusement all at the same time.

In the dark of the night, I hadn't pulled out my clear minty Burt's Bees lip balm, but instead the exact same shaped tube of dark berry tinted lip balm I had in my purse. Remember how I took full advantage of the moistening opportunity, rubbing it all around my lips and surrounding skin in a circular motion??? Well, I did a number on myself...I looked like a clown!

Sometimes, I still laugh so hard I can barely tell this story to others. It made perfect sense why people seemed a bit off at the grocery store that night; they weren't used to talking with a clown. As embarrassing as it might have been I owned the situation and I encourage you to do the same. Feel free to laugh at yourself and be okay when others join you. It's what makes the world go around, and you're creating health and happiness along the way.

CHAPTER 23

Creating Your New Normal

It's interesting to me how if one area of life is unraveling, it often feeds into another doing the same. I am not the queen of processes, but I've always enjoyed structure. In the days when my health was unraveling, it seemed the rest of my world was too. Take for instance how refreshed you feel after you kick off the morning with a shower and get dressed for the day. This simple act will set you in motion to tackle whatever the day holds. It seems so simple, cleaning up with a quick shower, but it truly felt like torture when I was in severe pain, and lacking the energy to stand long enough to do so. Often, I didn't shower until evening when I could go directly to sleep afterward. Therefore, my day was never really set in motion, by the lack of this one simple act. Once I started feeling healthy again, I got back into my routine and felt much more accomplished as a result. Sometimes it's just taking the one small step that will help you gain momentum to accomplish the rest of your goals for the day.

Structure

Structure creates a healthy environment for kids and adults alike. Think back on this past week; which days were you most productive, and which days did you feel frazzled and out of sorts? I'm confident that the days you had a plan, activities mapped out and a to-do list in hand, you were most productive whether at home, work, or play.

My life always seems to run more smoothly when I have my act together. Backpacks ready to go, lunches prepped, and all my work stuff waiting to head out the door with me. This leaves me enough time in the morning to get a quick workout in, spend extra time with the kids, or make a fancy breakfast for the family.

Then there are the days where one child can't find their left shoe while the other is crying because they lost their homework project. Life is not off to a good start on these days...

The whole point of creating structure is to ease stress in our lives and create health. I'll be the first one to tell you that I get bored after a while and sometimes like flying by the seat of my pants! However, there are plenty of areas of life where structure is necessary because the benefits are far too good. We'll cover a few of them in this chapter. Find ways to create structure in your life to support your health and happiness, and enjoy it when those fun spontaneous events happen. This offers you the best of both worlds.

The challenge with structure is keeping up with it, even when you're tired of doing so. Here are easy and effective tips to help you build structure for yourself and your family. You'll feel better for it and love what it provides you!

✖ **EXERCISE:** *Building Structure in Your Life*

1. First: Identify three areas in your life where structure is needed right now but doesn't really exist.

    1. _____

    2. _____

    3. _____

2. What is the consequence of not having structure in these three areas of your life? Are you tired, irritable, rushed, and worried?

_____

_____

_____

_____

_____

_____

_____

_____

_____

3. Now, let's look at just one area out of the three. What boundaries are necessary for you to provide structure in this area? Are you tired every morning because you stay up too late watching TV or catching up on all your Facebook messages? If this is the case, then you'll need to set a boundary for yourself around TV and computer time. No technology after 8 p.m. This gives you ample time to prep for bed and quietly read, meditate, pray, or breathe before heading into sound sleep for the night. If you're asleep by 10 p.m. and up at 6 a.m. then you're doing pretty well!

What boundaries are necessary for you to provide structure in this area?

_____

_____

_____

_____

_____

_____

Set your healthy boundaries and stick to them. As you observe what takes place in your life as a result of this new structure, take time to celebrate the positive change and express gratitude for your effort and focus.

4. Jot down what this structure provided you. Were you more productive in the day, hopping out of bed with energy in the morning, or better able to focus and stay on task? Whatever it provided you, write it down and express gratitude for this positive change in your life.

_____

_____

_____

_____

_____

_____

5. When the time comes that you make a poor choice or go back to your old ways—yes, this will happen because you are human—be kind to yourself. Recognize the consequence and readjust to get back into healthy choices. We learn from every choice, every circumstance, and every experience in our lives. There is no need to beat yourself up or feel guilty or upset. This is your time to shine; you're growing and expanding. If we were all perfect, life would be quite boring and we'd never grow beyond where we are today. So, celebrate the times that you make a choice you're not so pleased with, not because it wasn't a great choice but because you've recognized that you want to function differently, and you're learning and taking steps to do just that.

6. Making life change takes time. Practice providing structure consistently, over time so it becomes second nature. Be patient with the process and be kind to yourself every step of the way.

What's Your New "Normal"?

I had been through multiple personal trainers, educating one after another about my autoimmune and neuromuscular disease, and each failed me miserably. They would work my body so far beyond its limit that it'd take me weeks to recover.

And then I met Jeff.

I shared my concerns over the phone with Jeff during our introductory call, and he asked a bit about my disease. A day or two later I showed up for our in-person meeting to discuss teaming up for fitness; I about fell off my stool when he opened the file folder he had in his hand. He had researched all he could on mitochondrial myopathy and autoimmune disease and had printed information. He shared he'd never trained anyone with my specific condition but told me he felt confident he could get the job done. I was absolutely delighted and ready for my first session a few days later.

We were shooting for 30-minute workouts; keeping in mind that my body had had minimal physical activity for a few years leading up to our first session, along with the obvious complication of disease. I warmed up by walking on the treadmill and then we did some stretches on the mat for about 10 minutes. I thought this was the warm-up until Jeff said, "Great job today, that's a wrap and I'll see you on Thursday." What?? I was ticked. There was no way 15 minutes of walking and stretching constituted a workout. My mind went into competitive overdrive, envisioning the women I had seen when I first walked into the gym. They were boxing with Jeff as part of their training as I warmed up on the treadmill. I showed up on Thursday and it was the same thing. I was almost in tears as I shared with Jeff that I didn't feel like it was a workout at all.

Jeff helped me realize that this was the structure my body needed in that moment and reminded me I should be celebrating my effort. The 15 minute workouts grew to 30 minutes, and after a year I was training for hour-long sessions. I am so grateful for Jeff's structured guidance in helping me create a new normal and I'm excited for you to do the same! Enjoy creating your new normal with exercise, sleep, and more as you work through the following exercises.

Healthy Exercise

Exercise is probably one of the most challenging things for people to consistently include in their lives. It requires planning, scheduling and execution, and for whatever reason a lot of other things tend to take priority over 30 minutes (or more) of daily activity.

Research tells us that people who exercise tend to live longer, suffer less disease, sleep better, and maintain a healthy weight. So why not make exercise a priority in your life and make it your new "normal"?

While I'm not an expert in exercise training, I can help you identify your roadblocks and create a plan worth executing. Grab your pencil and take a few minutes to complete the following journal exercise.

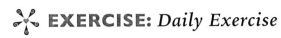 **EXERCISE:** *Daily Exercise*

The top three things that hold me back from completing my 30 minutes of daily activity are: (Think outside of the box on this one. Do you have fear about group exercise classes? Has it been so long since exercising that you don't even know where to start? Do you lack the energy to exercise?)

1. _____

2. _____

3. _____

Now let's explore how you feel when you do get daily movement and exercise.

When I exercise I feel:

1. _____
2. _____
3. _____

What roadblocks keep you from accomplishing daily exercise? Please consider your schedule, time, confidence, expectations, etc. and identify two things you must do to make room for daily exercise.

I need to do the following two things to make room for daily movement and exercise:

1. _____
2. _____

There are many exercise options available: yoga, outdoor sports, group classes, biking and hiking.

I'm most interested in trying the following types of exercise:

1. _____

   _____

2. _____

   _____

3. _____

   _____

Accountability is always helpful and research shows that partners who exercise together are more consistent with daily exercise than those who choose to go it alone. Find family, friends, or neighbors who might be interested in partnering up for exercise. If you do choose to go it alone, be sure to select an accountability partner to report in to for best success. Be sure this accountability partner will be supportive and a positive influence in your journey.

I plan to share my exercise goals with the following person(s) for weekly check-ins and support:

_____

_____

Be clear about the benefits you'd feel by including 30 minutes of exercise into your daily schedule, and commit to your new exercise plan today. Create your new "normal" by outlining your exercise plan in the chart below. Once finished, you'll need to schedule time in your calendar to execute the plan and follow through.

I commit to making the following exercise plan my new "normal":

New Normal Exercise Plan

Monday	Tuesday	Wednesday	Thursday	Friday	Saturday	Sunday

I commit to this new "normal" today! I am confident that I will stick to it, create health and happiness and feel great as a result.

Cheers to my fitness, my health, and my happiness,

_____

Your Name Here

Now throw your gym shoes on and start living your new "normal." The life you desire is right there waiting for you; commit to your plan, share your goals, believe in yourself, and make it happen.

Sleep Like a Baby

When was the last time you sacked out and woke up feeling refreshed and energized? I hope your answer is just last night...and every night for that matter. Unfortunately, most Americans don't remember the last time they felt this way.

In my opinion, in order to sleep like a baby we need to treat ourselves like a baby.

Structure: Have a set bedtime every night so things stay consistent. The average adult needs 7-8 hours of consistent shut-eye in order to be most productive, and feel well. This means heading to bed around 10 p.m. every night and waking around 6 a.m.

Got kids? Children should be provided the following according to the National Sleep Foundation:

- Newborns: Sleep in irregular patterns anywhere from 10.5-18 hours per day
- 3-11 months: 9-12 hours every night plus 2-4 naps during the day
- 1-3 years: 12-14 hours of sleep in a 24 hour period (including naps)
- 3-5 years: 11-13 hours every night
- 5-12 years: 10-11 hours every night

Avoid Caffeine: Just as we wouldn't feed our children caffeine, especially right before bed, we should honor the same for ourselves. If you do choose to drink caffeine in the day it is best to stop all caffeine after 2 p.m. This will give your body enough time to process the caffeine before you head off to sleep.

Quiet Time: Most often, children have a bedtime routine which includes all the proper cleaning of food from the face, teeth brushing, a trip to the potty, and a sweet bed-time story. You'll notice there was no "checking email, texting, or working on the computer" included in the routine. Keep your routine as clean as a child's routine. Shut down all technology and phones at least one hour before heading to bed in order to achieve optimal sleep. Take an hour of time before bed to relax, listen to classical music, read, journal about your day, or spend time with your significant other.

Eat Well: We all need three balanced meals a day, and maybe a snack here and there. I can't imagine sitting my children down to a big meal at eight at night and then sending them right off to bed. As adults, especially if we're entertaining or out with clients, we tend to eat large meals loaded with excess fat and salt, etc. late at night. The purpose of sleep is to allow the body to repair and replenish. Your blood is purified, your liver detoxifies the body, and all your organs are resetting for another day. The body needs to be able to focus all of its energy on this, so when you have food in the gut that needs to be digested, the body will give up some of its "repair" energy for the needed digestion. Make breakfast and lunch your biggest meals and go light for dinner. As a rule, all meals should be consumed three hours before bed. If you need a light snack before bed, eat an hour before you go to sleep. Some foods known to aid in sleep are: oats, bananas, tart cherries or tart cherry juice, and almonds.

Eat, Play, Sleep: If you've read a book about raising a child it may have included the theory of "eat, play, sleep." This routine ensures that your child has structure in the day and gets plenty of activity before nap and bedtime. We need the same in our lives. Activity is important for sleep, as well as play! Be sure to get up from the desk, take a walk and get fresh air. Accomplish 30 minutes of exercise every day and schedule "play time" into your calendar. Think about the activities you loved to do as a child and start incorporating some of that same activity in your life today. There's no age limit for playing in the sandbox.

Remember that we have a choice in every matter, including sleep. Make small changes so you eventually achieve your sleep goals. If you head to bed at midnight every night, you surely won't be able to switch to a 10 p.m. bedtime right away. Start small and build up. Go to bed at 11:45 p.m. for a few nights, then move it up to 11:30 p.m. and continue moving up by 15-min increments until you reach your 10 p.m. goal. The pay-off is huge; you'll feel better physically and emotionally and you're most productive and happy when you're adequately refreshed and energized.

❈ EXERCISE: *Sleep*

In order to achieve adequate sleep and support my body in health I will do the following:

Happy snoozing!

Structure can provide ease, predictability, and support us in health. But it doesn't mean we can't fit in quick bursts of healthy fun on the fly! This rule applies to table food and life food. You can spend all day creating a gourmet meal, or in a pinch make a protein and veggie wrap accompanied by a side salad and get the same amount of nutrition from each. It's about using your time and energy most wisely to achieve the outcome you desire. Some of the tips I share in the next chapter will give you opportunity for quick, healthy activities to support you in your goal of healthy, vibrant living.

CHAPTER 24

Small Dose of Goodness

This chapter is loaded with quick, healthy activities that will help you feel better in an instant. The next 15 minute break you take from your workspace will never be the same; and just wait to see what you can do with the gift of breath to ease stress and bring balance to your day. The section on the 3 F's that follows is a fun one; something we all need to consider but rarely do. Cleaning your closet may not seem to fit into "quick healthy activities" but it opens up possibility and you're going to feel a huge weight roll off your shoulders when you do the exercise. It's time to feel fabulous in an instant.

Healthy Things to Do in 15 Minutes or Less

Picture this...You're on a mission, glued to the computer screen and determined to get your project completed by your 3 p.m. deadline. The problem is your brain is in overload, your back is aching from sitting so long, and your stomach is rumbling because you forgot to eat lunch. NOW is the time to get up from the computer and take 15 minutes just for you! The health benefits will far outweigh the risk you may be taking by walking away from your computer;

you'll feel energized, renewed, refreshed, and ready to tackle the project that still awaits your attention.

Ideally, we should step away for multiple short breaks throughout the day. Be proactive about it and you'll consistently feel more positive energy and calm in your day.

Here's a list of healthy things you can do to fill the 15 minute break:

1. Step outside for a 15-minute brisk walk (you'll walk 2,000 steps!).
2. Hit the stairwell for a good climb.
3. Make yourself a cup of hot green tea.
4. Complete a circuit (or two) of push-ups, sit-ups, tricep dips, and jumping jacks.
5. Find some fresh air and give a friend a call.
6. In need of a laugh? Pull up some comedy clips on YouTube and get your laugh on!
7. Enjoy a light snack of homemade trail mix.
8. Refill your water bottle and drink half of it.
9. Stretch your muscles.
10. Take deep breaths and release all the tension you feel with each out breath.
11. Sit in the sun, close your eyes, listen to nature, and be present.
12. Smell the flowers.
13. Read a quick article from your favorite magazine.
14. Write down 10 things you're grateful for today.
15. Savor a piece of rich, dark chocolate and tell yourself that all is well; in the end it will all get done.

As I've said before, we have a choice in every matter. Choose to step away from the desk, choose to enjoy a quiet moment to yourself every evening, and choose to live in a healthy, vibrant way. Your body and mind will love you for it.

Quiet Time and Space

We rarely get a moment of space and quiet unless we make the effort to create it in our day. Taking time to quiet the brain, connect with nature and create space for your own self love and care can feel impossible but it's absolutely necessary to implement for our health and happiness. We tend to rush through the day, running here, there and everywhere, and we end up exhausted.

Our days are full of family duties, work obligations, and the general busyness of life. We often feel our productivity comes from crossing off the items on the to-do list, and we find ourselves doing things we really don't care to do. The truth is, life on Earth is a brief gift, and our time is too precious to be used like this. If we want our lives to be balanced and healthy, we need to lessen our load and increase our time for self-care. This means planning less in a day, and prioritizing those things that make our hearts sing. If we must accomplish many things each day, we can still change the quality with which we complete the tasks. Taking even brief moments in the day to relax and breathe, or stepping outside to take in the fresh air, can reduce stress and provide you a renewed outlook for the day.

Belly breathing is an easy, transportable, simple task that can turn your outward thoughts to a moment of inward thinking, increase your body awareness, and provide you the opportunity to get in touch with your inner voice. When we rush through our days, we are inundated with outside noise, emotion, tension, and situations that can cause anxiety, chaos, and stress in our body. This is the type of activity that leads to disease in the body followed by aches and pain, fatigue, and other symptomology.

Join me for this exercise. Envision your belly as a balloon. The goal is to fill up every space of that balloon with air. Breathe in deeply and let your belly expand as a balloon would. When you get to the "fill" line, take one more deep breath and pause. Now release all the air from the belly, deflating every bit of the balloon. When you get to the final little space of air, blow out one extra breath. Repeat this cycle of breathing for one minute. Relax your shoulders and neck, take in the positive energy of this moment and connect with yourself.

You should feel differently now than before you did the exercise. In one minute you can feel relaxed, calm the stress response in your body, connect with your inner voice and focus on positive thoughts and affirmation to carry you through the day. Simple. Effective. Transportable. Necessary.

Every one of us can find one minute of time in the day, and if you're lucky maybe one minute every hour. Do this for yourself. Make the time to belly breathe, and as you continue your practice, move your time up by one minute every week until you hit the five-minute mark. These five minutes will be one of your most treasured, refreshing moments of the day.

�֎ EXERCISE: *Breathing (expanded)*

Find a quiet space for yourself. Sit and get comfortable. Close your eyes, relax your shoulders, roll your head in a relaxing circular motion to the right and then to the left. Place one hand on your heart and breathe deeply in through your nose then exhale through the mouth. While continuing this breathing pattern, recite a positive intention on the in-breath and release the negativity in your life with each exhale. Focus on what you need at this time for your positive affirmation; if you're struggling with self-confidence you might say something like "I am enough," if you're worrying about something out of your control, you can recite "All is well in this life."

Speak your affirmation clearly and confidently as if you already feel it and believe it. On the exhale, release the negativity that exists: "I release the need for control," "I release all negativity," or "I release all fear." One affirmation with each inhale and one focused release with each exhale. This exercise is especially helpful in moments of anxiousness. You'll enter your day with clarity and calm, and when you repeat this exercise before slumber it'll support you in calm, sound sleep.

The 3 F's: Fit, Flatter, Feel like a Million Bucks

1. Fit
2. Flatter
3. Feel like a million bucks!

These 3 F's are the key to cleaning your closet. You might wonder how cleaning the closet lands itself in a book about creating health. In my humble opinion, the more we purge the unnecessary from our lives, the more room we'll have for new opportunity, joy, and health to enter. How many articles of clothing are sitting in your closet right now, never being worn, because they don't meet the 3 F's?

Our closets need a little cleansing, just like our own body system! I challenge you to take time over the next two weeks to purge and gift your local thrift shop with the items that would fit, flatter, and make another individual feel like a million bucks. You can do it all at once, or take 15 minutes once a week for a mini refresher. Here are some guidelines to help you purge in quick fashion:

Fit:

We all know what a nice fitting pair of pants and shirt looks like on us. Find what works for you, provides comfort, and can be worn all day without experiencing symptoms like blistering, restricting, chafing, or riding (you know what I mean). It's not worth it! Your clothes should fit comfortably, and you should feel comfortable in them; no readjusting, pulling and tugging necessary.

Flatter:

Know your body type and love every bit of it! There is clothing to flatter each of us. I tend to go for A-line skirts and V-neck tops because they work well for me. What works best for you? If you don't know what your body type is, or what clothes will be most flattering, explore articles on line, reach out to a stylist at your favorite store or bring the friend that will tell all on your next shopping trip. There are plenty of times where an outfit looks perfect on my friend, and when I try something similar on it simply doesn't work for me; the outfit is not as flattering because I have a different body type than my friend. No need for wishing for something different in these scenarios. While we can all work to gain more muscle tone and better support the body we've been given, we need to love every bit of ourselves along the way and find the clothes that flatter us right here and now. Gentlemen, while you're not reaching for the A-line skirt as I am, there's plenty for you to consider here as well. There are many styles of pants and shirts available, relaxed fit, slim fit, flat front, and more. Find the style that flatters your body type; play around with fit, color and patterns to find what flatters you most and get rid of the items in your closet that don't align with your findings.

Feel like a million bucks!

Stop waiting to lose the last five pounds, or waiting for the "right time" to find clothes that make you feel like a million bucks. The time is now! When you feel good in the clothes you wear, it does something for your energy and spirit. You truly feel alive when you feel good about your appearance. The clothes don't need to cost an arm and leg, or necessarily follow the current trends; they just need to make YOU feel like a million bucks. If they don't, you'll find them taking space in your closet and never wearing them. This is a waste of money, space, and energy that could be spent on more productive things.

EXERCISE: *Cleanse the Closet*

It's time for a little fun; this is an exercise the whole family can do to feel healthier in an instant.

Take Action:
- *Set 30-60 minutes of time aside to purge your closet.*
- *Take all the clothes from your closet and place them on your bed.*
- *One by one, sort through the articles of clothing, trying them on if necessary to see if they meet the 3 F's. You may already know some that don't; there's no need to try these on.*
- *Stop dawdling; you're on the clock and you're getting the job done in quick fashion.*
- *After trying on the article of clothing, you either put it in the giveaway pile, or hang/fold it to be returned to your closet.*
- *At the end of your purge, bag the pile of donation clothes and put the rest away in your closet. You now have a wardrobe full of clothes that flatter and make you feel like a million bucks.*
- *Congratulations! Now put the donation bag in the car and motor over to the donation center; you're going to make a lot of people happy today.*
- *If you have another closet in your home, you can set time aside and repeat these steps.*

In very little time, you can give yourself a quick, healthy burst of goodness! You too can come up with fun things to do in 15 minutes or less. Start doing sit-ups on each commercial break, park as far away as you can in the parking lot, or have a dance party with your grandkids! The options are endless.

CHAPTER 25

Believe It Can Be

It seems crazy to me that one act could've caused me so much angst when it came to believing in myself, but all too often this is how the self-doubt begins.

I was in the concert choir in high school and training to perform at the Solo & Ensemble Festival. This is a large event where many schools come together to compete. My aunt, who is a music teacher, worked for hours with me to perfect my piece and prepare me for success.

We had finished our competition as a choir, and my solo performance was to take place a couple of hours thereafter. My nerves were building as the minutes ticked by. The performers from my school had supported all the other choir members who performed solos throughout the day, and my performance would close out the competition. As I was talking to my mom, we noticed everyone gathering their belongings. The choir director walked over and shared that he decided it'd been a long day, and he was going to get everyone back to the school. The bus would be leaving without me, and he asked my mom if she'd be okay taking me home. We had no choice but to say yes, and off they went.

When the time came, I walked in and stood in front of the judges. My heart beat out of my chest, and my mind was in a million different places about why they'd leave me when everyone else was supported. Maybe I wasn't good enough, or worthy of support. It didn't matter how many loving and kind words my mom shared with me; the belief I had in myself had been shredded into small remnants, barely visible to the naked eye. As for the competition, I'd say I bombed it.

That feeling of standing in front of the judges stayed with me for the longest time. I continued to sing long after high school, but felt sick every time beforehand worrying about failure. I didn't want to bomb like I had in the competition; self-doubt was strong and I was incredibly self-conscious until one specific event: my own wedding. I had planned to surprise my husband and sing for him in our ceremony. The song was Valentine, by Martina McBride. The same feelings of fear rose up inside of me as the time drew near, and then calm, like I've never experienced before, washed over me as I took my husband's hands, turned to him and began to sing. In that moment, he was the only thing that existed, and I remember feeling unconditionally loved. It was the first time I sang freely, without hesitation, without worry about what others might think or say; it was amazing!

I share this with you because it's important for us to realize our ability, to embrace every bit of who we are, and believe in ourselves to the fullest extent. The grandest of all loves is to be able to love yourself unconditionally; when you do there'll be nothing to stop you. No opinions, comments, or critical thoughts to consume you. Because you'll be confident in yourself, your gifts, your ability to love and all that you offer this world, by simply being you.

One other consideration is that people do the best they can with the tools they've been given. In the moment of the bus leaving, I felt betrayed, unworthy, and humiliated. Looking back, I don't believe my choir director had any intention of making me feel this way. We read into things, and respond in various ways because of our belief systems, events in life, and how we've been conditioned. Had I been able to separate myself from the situation, there may have been a different outcome. The thoughts of unworthiness, betrayal, and humiliation were subconscious thoughts driving my feelings.

When you find yourself in a challenging situation, and self-doubt starts creeping in, I want you to ask yourself one quick question: "Would I ever consciously choose to feel this way?" If the answer is no, it's a good indication that your thoughts and feelings are being driven by the subconscious mind. Tap into the feelings you're having and then explore how you'd consciously choose to feel in the situation. Focus on these positive, conscious feelings and allow yourself to move forward.

Loving yourself unconditionally and providing others the permission to react as they desire will free you beyond measure. This was a very big part of my journey back to health; as much as the table food was doing to heal my body, my thoughts were equally powerful. My health crisis helped me realize that my life food was just as out of balance as my table food. My sugar addiction was being fed just as much as my need for approval. Start observing these patterns in your own life as you journey through this chapter. I'm so excited for you and proud of the work you're doing for yourself.

Believe!

Belief plays a big role in healing and health. How we choose to communicate this belief with our own selves, and others, can impact us positively or negatively depending on the route we take. Prior to being ill, friends and coworkers would describe me as "always positive" or comment that I could always see the glass half full. But I must say something drastically shifted for me through the days of deterioration.

For almost two years there were a lot of new symptoms popping up one after another, and my body seemed to ebb and flow with its ability to function. Living in a body full of pain, fatigue, nausea, headaches, and sadness is daunting, to say the least. On a great day, I might make it up to school to volunteer in my daughter's class for an hour, and on a bad day I barely got by just tending to normal daily tasks to care for my children. The unpredictability was tough to handle, and often left me feeling depressed and isolated. I was doing my due diligence, seeing one doctor after another, but would return home without answers time and time again. Unfortunately, my belief system was challenged. I didn't begin to change until a few months after my diagnosis, when I decided that I no longer wanted to figure out how to die gracefully; I was going to choose to live.

The Power of Positive Thinking, a book read by over five million people since Norman Vincent Peale first published it in 1952, was a launching pad for me. One of the toughest challenges I had, coming off the diagnosis of a rare neuromuscular disease that would take my life, was sleeping. I would be so gripped with fear each night as I lay in bed that my sleep was restless. Worries of the days to come, how my children would cope with my deterioration, what this would hold for my marriage, and more, consumed my mind. This was all until I decided to recite positive affirmations and supportive biblical versus as I fell into slumber. It may seem a simple act, but it was life changing for me. For the first time in a long while I found myself feeling glimmers of hope.

Belief means having confidence, faith, and trust in something greater than ourselves. It sometimes means taking a leap of faith. It's trusting in the path that you're on, knowing that you'll grow and expand with your journey. Belief does not mean that everything will go just as we want it to go. Or be just as we want it to be. Rather, it provides us a sound place to find our calm, believe in the power that exists far beyond us, and create ways to work with whatever our situation may be.

It took me a good six years to fully believe that my body was capable of healing, and trust that it could function at a high level. Even though my health was improving, my great days would often be followed by challenging ones in the first few years of the healing process. When I felt great and saw that my body was getting back to normal functioning I was full of belief that anything was possible, and that the dark days were behind me. Then, inevitably, I would push myself too far, beyond the healthy boundaries of my body's needs, and immediately start to feel symptomatic in one way or another. When this cycle happened, I would instantly be triggered back into the place of fear and anger. Anger at my body for its inability to stay healthy, and fear of how things might progress. But over the years, what I've realized is that this is not a healthy relationship for me and my body to have. Who can grow and flourish in an environment of fear and anger? No one. This realization caused me to change how I speak to, care for, and support my body. It also greatly impacted my belief system.

Take a moment and picture a small child you know and love. He or she is about five years old, always full of energy, ready to conquer the world with creativity and the belief that everything is possible. Now, imagine yourself saying these words to the small child, in a loud, angry voice. "You are pathetic!" "How could you do this to me?" "Why would you betray me?" "How could you let me down like this?" "How am I supposed to love you when all you do is cause me pain?" "I hate you!"

These awful and harmful words are the words I used to speak to my body. I hated what it was doing to me, and couldn't find a way to love it unconditionally. Speaking to your body is like speaking to a small child. It is my hope that you'll never speak to the child you know and love in the manner I shared. It would scar them for life, and create such feelings of hurt and unworthiness that they may never function at their full potential. The body is no different. If you want it to reach its full potential, you need to speak to it kindly and treat it with love and care.

The body speaks to us each and every day; a small sniffle, a crazy headache, pain, and more. Most often, we rush through our day and not even give it a second thought. Our symptoms become annoyances, things we just don't have time for. If it were the same small child you pictured speaking to you, sharing that they have an awful headache, you'd pause, inquire more and if needed seek medical attention. The symptoms we feel are the body's way of communicating there is a problem.

It's time to believe that our body is there for us, to grow, heal, do well, and support us in our goals and dreams. But in order for it to function at its best, it needs a lot of TLC. It's time to change your beliefs, and understand that you have the choice to love and care for your body just as you would a small child. Listen to it speak to you, explore what it needs from you, and give it as much support as you can. Believe that anything is possible, and find ways to love yourself and your body regardless of the situation.

We can choose to have a positive outlook, a belief that even though life may look differently than before a diagnosis, there is possibility and so much we CAN do. You'll experience symptoms throughout life, sometimes a flare up of an old challenge, or something completely new. When this occurs, take time to acknowledge what's happening and ensure that you're supporting your body the best you know how. Silently let it know through messages such as, "Thank you for speaking to me today; I feel my swollen joints and am doing everything I can to support you. We'll figure this out." This is a much more loving, positive way to build a relationship with your body.

Believe in yourself, in your body's ability to thrive, and in the greatness of God and his entire universe. If there are days when it's too much to bear, ask for guidance and strength and call on your loved ones to help fill a need. Believe that your choice matters and that you can participate in life as you wish.

�֎ EXERCISE: *Belief and the Body*

What does your relationship with your body look like today?

_____

_____

_____

_____

_____

_____

_____

_____

How do you connect with your belief in something greater than yourself? This can be through prayer, meditation, community groups, and more. As a beautiful mentor of mine always says, connect with God, the Universe, or whatever it is that you believe makes the sun shine and the grass grow.

How can you create a more loving relationship with your body?

How can you best support the needs of your body at this time?

How could you enhance your belief system and nourish your faith?

_____

_____

_____

_____

_____

_____

_____

What one simple verse or positive affirmation could you recite daily to support you through challenging days?

_____

_____

_____

_____

_____

_____

_____

CHAPTER 26

Love

Love is a beautiful gift to be shared with all; including the one and only, incredible YOU! Love means many things to many people; to me it means celebration, healing, forgiveness, joy, unconditional care, peace, and a feeling greater than anything else I know. God is love.

As I write this, it's June 23rd, 2016; it's been just over nine years since my health crisis began. Sometimes it feels like a lifetime ago, and other days it feels less so. I am thankful for each and every step of this journey, because I've learned something each step of the way. What I've realized through the years is that love is at the center; every lesson, every triumph, the whole transformation. The healthy boundaries, healthy food, healthy relationships; they all begin and end with self-love and care.

"It's No Business of Mine What You Think About Me"

There's only so much time in the day and so much worrying you can take on before you become all consumed with other peoples' thoughts about you. As a young woman, I didn't understand the concept of loving myself for who I was. Nor did I understand that I was divinely designed to just be me. Instead, I was consumed with the need to please others, and regardless of the type of interaction (with friends, family, co-workers) I would spend too much time re-playing scenarios and wondering if I said and did the right thing, worrying about the impression I left on someone. Wondering what I could I have changed, how I should interact in the future, and on and on. It's tiring even recalling all of this! Maybe you can relate. As much as I worried about what others thought about me, the bigger fact of the matter is that I wasn't sure of myself. The biggest issue for any of us in this scenario is the fear of how WE will react, what WE may think about ourselves, as a result of the response that oth-ers have towards us.

A great example of this is public speaking. I happily get up in front of hundreds of people and share an inspiring story, or talk about nutrition and life fulfillment. Out of these hundreds of peo-ple, there will be some who will have critical thoughts about me. Maybe they think I'm too thin, maybe they don't like how I talk, maybe they don't care at all about what I have to say, or maybe they simply hate my outfit. Whatever the case, I will never please every-one. I could take these comments or the looks that people give, try to change myself, and go back to the old days of wondering "what if?" Or I can choose differently.

Focus on loving yourself for who you are. Share your gifts, and emit the positive energy you wish to receive. With a little bit of work, we can all find it, cherish it and celebrate it. When you love every bit of yourself, focus on sharing your amazing gifts, and honor yourself in health, it won't matter what others have to say about you. There will always be an opinion, a criticism, a look passed your way. Take a deep breath, connect with the amazing person you are, feed this thought with positive words of encouragement, and understand that those opinions, criticisms, and looks are their business and not yours.

Stay in your happy, loving place, whether you're honoring your new eating habits, saying no for the first time, or giving permission for another person to have the opinion they want to have. Love resides within you, embrace it and know you're perfect just as you are.

Giving Love

This moment is clear as day; I had known my husband for only three months. He was visiting his parents in Michigan and I had flown to San Diego to complete the first Rock-n-Roll marathon to support Leukemia Team in Training. It was the night before the race, and I had called to say hello. He was at a dinner and his parent's voicemail came on. I shared my excitement about the race and that I was looking forward to talking with him and then paused at the end of the voicemail before saying goodbye. I paused because I was going to say "I love you" and then realized that this voicemail would be played aloud, as it was many years ago when the answering machine was just that, a machine. My voice would ring through the house as the play button was pushed. I felt self-conscious about expressing my love for this man in front of others. I wasn't sure what his response would be; we had already said these words to one another, but hadn't shouted it from the rooftops.

When he called later that night, he said in his sweet, calm voice that he knew I had wanted to say "I love you" during the stillness of the pause. He read my mind, and knew my words even when they weren't spoken. I regretted that moment of pause for a long time and decided then and there that I would give my love as often as I could, sharing these three words with family and with friends.

In time, I realized there was one other place I could express my love for the betterment of my health and healing, and that was the love and gratitude I have for my body and all it provides me. Positive self-talk and love will help you own your power, brighten your day, and heal the body. I've seen it work time and time again.

Give love a try! Next time you throw on an outfit for your date night, or a fine suit for your presentation at work, give yourself some loving self-talk. "Dang, I'm rockin' this dress," or "I'm confident and strong" leading into the presentation. Give of yourself to others in loving ways, by sharing a heart-felt compliment, telling the person how much they mean to you, and giving your full time and attention to a conversation. Remember to give the same gift of love to yourself. When your thoughts, behaviors, and actions come from a place of love, your mindset shifts, your health improves, and the one thing you thought impossible starts to feel possible. Love is everywhere within you and around you. See it, participate in it, share it and revel in it. It's yours for the giving and taking.

❧ EXERCISE: *The LOVE Exercise*

For the next seven days make it your mission to give the gift of love to yourself and one other person each day. Feel free to be an over-achiever here, and spread more love if you'd like. It's only going to enhance your journey and health.

Write down seven areas of your life that you'll focus on in your self-love portion of the exercise. These areas might include appearance, patience, confidence, or expectations.

1._____
2._____
3._____

4._____
5._____
6._____
7._____

Now, write down the names of seven people you'd like to gift your love to in the coming week:

1._____
2._____
3._____
4._____
5._____
6._____
7._____

Observe what happens over the next seven days. When you live and work from a place of love, love tends to surround you and chances are you're going to feel it happen. Be open to all that life and love has in store for you.

CHAPTER 27

Love Life, Feel Vibrant, Be Healthy

B efore you venture into this last chapter, I'd like you to flip back to the beginning of the book. Find the letter you wrote to your body and reread it now. Connect with how you felt at the time. Review the goals you shared, and read about the relationship you'd like to have with your body. You may have new thoughts after working through the exercises and information in this book; that's to be expected. It's also good to see where you started. Feel free to add to your letter, or write a second letter to your body and share your thoughts about moving forward together in this journey.

This is your time to shine, to build the life you desire and deserve, and be the best you can in health and happiness. You have everything you need right inside of you to make it happen!

Building Your Team

Through the years of working with my failing body I realized that no one person could be everything to me. It didn't mean they didn't love me, or care about me, but rather it meant that we all have a different way of dealing with crisis, grief, fear, sadness, guilt, and more. Each person in my life was able to support me in a different way; for this I am forever grateful, because had it not been for this love and support I don't know if I'd be thriving like I am today.

There's so much emotion and so many unanswered questions when you experience a life-altering health event. My husband was the person who would hold me, let me cry, encourage me to find the positive and try new things. He was working full time; coming home to an unkempt house, he often had to make dinner and clean up, and help get our young children off to sleep for the night. He fell asleep next to a wife who mostly wept at night and would wake up to a wife in tears because her pain was too much to bear. What I never really thought about during that time was the fact that his social life dwindled, his ability to care for himself took a back seat, he was losing the wife he knew and loved and there simply was no more room left for him to manage anything else. He couldn't be the person I vented to about my pain, or about another failed doctor visit, or about any other negative thing I came up with (there was a lot). But he was always there, encouraging me, holding me through the tears and fighting to keep our family life pieced together.

I turned to my sisters for a lot of the venting, and would call on friends in time of need. Each of them offered something unique. My sister-in-law always level-headed to calm my frantic state, my friend Jess always there to share my tears, my friend Elayne seeking answers, and my sisters and brother a stronghold when I was falling apart. My parents and mother- and father-in-law would travel to visit and care for the kids in time of great need. There were many people who played a role in this journey; I could never express enough gratitude and thanks for all they've done.

You too need to build your team. In times of illness as well as health, a team is always necessary. Your team should include your health care professionals who help you proactively be well, the friends who share your similar interests, the person you can call and vent to, the shoulder to cry on, the people who make you laugh, the friends who can help with your kiddos, and your greatest love to share the journey with. You will be a player on others' teams as well. Learn from each of them, be your own advocate, and cherish the love, care, and guidance they offer you.

A lot of time and care has been spent throughout the past nine years to find doctors and holistic professionals who would work with me as a team, respect my need to advocate, ask questions and be a part of the solution. You'll find some professionals who value this, and honor your requests, and others who simply do not. Remember that you're hiring these professionals into your team to provide you the best care possible. Sometimes you may reach out in a proactive manner, and other times in a reactive manner because you may already be experiencing a health crisis. Either way, you are in charge of creating your team. Make sure you work with people you trust; ask as many questions as you'd like, and decide if they're the best fit for your needs. It may take time and effort, but it'll be well worth it to have a high-functioning team working to help you achieve long-term health.

Allow the people in your life to help you also; they'll love to do so. From meals being delivered to my door, to phone calls and care packages, people near and far helped me through my journey. There is no physical or emotional way for everyone to be everything to you, but collectively, they can. Pick up the phone, ask for support, and express your love and gratitude for their kindness. It does take a village, and for all the love, kindness, and grace I received I will be forever thankful. I know you'll feel the same!

The Power of Words

Music has always been a constant in my life. If you walk into my home on any given day, you'll hear tunes coming from one of my many Pandora stations. Depending on my mood and activity, you might sway to the beautiful sounds of George Winston, kick up your heels with a bit of country, or sing the night away with some of my favorite artists (there are too many to list here!).

There is one song, however, that can instantly take me back to a moment in time; a very difficult moment. The words spoke to me clearly as I lay in savasana. I had taken my first-ever yoga class and this is the song the instructor played for us while we lay still in the corpse pose. I was very ill at the time and attempting to get back into exercise. I was barely sleeping, had minimal energy in the day, my pain level was at an all-time high, and my muscles were weak at best. There were more difficult days than promising ones, and I was happy to be out trying something new. These are the words that filled my space as I lay there on the floor of the yoga room:

When you try your best but you don't succeed.
When you get what you want but not what you need.
When you're so tired but you can't sleep.
Stuck in reverse.
And the tears come streaming down your face.
When you lose something you can't replace.
When you love someone but it goes to waste,
Could it be worse?
Lights will guide you home
And ignite your bones
And I will try to fix you.

I heard these words and I lost all emotional control. The tears came streaming down my face; the yoga instructor walked over and gently placed a towel over my eyes. I was free to take part in this emotional release.

What I realized while lying there is the one I was losing was myself. My incredible body that had always been there for me was the thing that I couldn't replace. I was completely stuck; I had been trying my best to get answers and find someone to help me and was repeatedly let down. "I will try to fix you" played over and over in my mind. I knew then that I would never give up; it wasn't even an option. This was the moment I started to see my body in a new light and I began to give it the love it needed to thrive.

Chris Martin and the Coldplay band don't know the impact they've had on my life because of their emotional delivery of these words in song. Sometimes it's the small gifts in our day that light up our entire world with hope.

If you're in a place of suffering, grief, despair, fear, or hopelessness, it is my hope that you too may be blessed with the power of words. May you take flight and know that all things are possible, including the health of your body, mind, and spirit. Your body is beautifully and divinely designed. It wants to do well for you, heal, and be strong. Sometimes it takes a great deal of time to figure it out, sometimes the road to healing is very difficult physically and emotionally, and you may feel like giving up. That's the moment you breathe, and then breathe again. It's in the quiet space that you can connect to your heart, find peace in any moment, and know that you have it in you to continue the journey no matter how difficult the road may be. There is a beautiful gift in every life experience and while I couldn't see it for a very long time, it was there for me in the end. I wish you much love in your journey, blessings for the ability to see the good, and trust that in the end, there is beauty in all of it.

Be Your Own Advocate

In the beginning of this book, I asked you what you'd do if you had the opportunity to transform your life. If you've made it this far, it means you've grabbed hold of the opportunity, opened yourself to new ideas, and explored ways to enhance your health and happiness. While the book may have provided guidance along the way, YOU, my dear friend, are the sole person responsible for taking action.

Putting together your team, as I mentioned above, starts by being your own best advocate. By this, I mean taking charge, making decisions, and leading the way. In our society, it's common to rely on professionals for guidance, and follow their every word. But that's not always going to be in your best interest. You and only you know your body better than anyone else on this beautiful earth. You understand when something is off and you know how good you feel when you're functioning at your best. Being your own advocate means taking the necessary steps to stay healthy for the long haul. It's time you lead the team, provide input, share ideas and thoughts, and advocate for your health and wellbeing. There's a root cause to every issue in our body; a reason why something is breaking down, or changing. Be sure that you fight to know the cause of your ailing body, to understand the reasoning behind every procedure and prescription, and find a team of professionals who will work with you as a team.

If there's one final thought I can leave you with, it is this. We have a choice in every matter; please choose to actively participate in all aspects of your life.

In reflecting on my journey, I realize that I participated in all of it; the brain fog, the stomach aches, the fatigue, the despair, the weak muscles, and the many sleepless nights. In the thick of my ill days, I had no idea that my choices were causing harm and feeding disease in my body. It wasn't until much later that I realized my Life Food and Table Food choices were contributing to all of the illness I felt. It was a tough realization, because I was starting to understand the lack of awareness I had, and the thought of relearning everything was overwhelming. But I started, with one simple choice at a time, to change my life and I'm so happy that you're choosing to do the same!

As you participate in your journey, keep in mind the team you build may look different as you go through life. Over the years my team has consisted of medical doctors, holistic doctors, chiropractors, acupuncturists, energy healers, and others. I've been able to explore lots of different teachings, modalities, and experiences, and each has provided a benefit to me along the way. Find what works for you, explore new options if you aren't making the headway you expected to make, know that your body wants to do well for you; and believe that in time you'll find exactly what you need.

Navigating the journey of a failing body can be interesting at times. I learned that when someone says "How are you today?" they're most often looking for the surface, "I'm doing just fine," answer. Most often, when I did share the truth about how I was doing, it was too overwhelming to hear. Because my body was in a difficult place, my thoughts were too and I would often talk about the pain, fatigue, and hurt I was experiencing. In time, I kept guarded with this information, and put on the happy face. While it wasn't what I really wanted to do, it served the situation best. I share this with you because the lesson I took away from it is that we all go through challenging times in life. We never know what someone is going through on any given day. Please provide patience, give a listening ear when you ask someone how they're doing, and if you'd like, you can say a silent blessing for the person who's having a rough day.

Your kindness will help them get through the rest of their day, and add a little sunshine to their life.

It's time now to consider everything you've learned, select the tools and strategies that will serve you best at this time in your life, and run with them! Refer back anytime you want to explore a topic in greater depth. We also have resources on the website. In order to feel good and look good for life, you'll need to continue implementing the tips and strategies outlined here on a regular basis. The book is your guide—that's it. Take initiative every day to take one simple step forward and make health happen!

Remember to follow the rules I shared with you in the beginning of the book:

- To yourself you must be true; take responsibility for all you do.
- Be open to new possibilities, ideas and thoughts.
- Respect all the emotions that surface during your journey.
- Release the need to control the responses of others.
- Above all, always be kind to YOU.

You're precious, and talented, and divinely designed to rock this world simply by being YOU. So go be your amazing self. Give to yourself and others, share your gifts, and create health and happiness each and every day. You can do it: I'm cheering you on every step of the way!

XO,

Angela

Acknowledgements

It takes a village to create a book. While my two hands may have scribed the words that cover the pages of this manuscript, there were far more people involved in the creation of it. For their love, support, hard work, and encouragement I am forever grateful.

To Rob, Tori and Sean: Thank you for blessing me with your grace, never-ending support and the many, many hugs along the way. There's no greater love to be had in my life than the three of you. xoxoxo

Thank you to my family and friends for all the kind words of encouragement, support from near and far, and shared excitement every step of the way. Much love and gratitude to all of you!

To the amazing team who helped me bring this book to life, my brilliant editor Alexandra O'Connell and remarkable designers Paul Vorreiter and Michelle White.

Dr. AJ Christoff, Dr. Stephen Smith and Dr. Laura Larson, thank you for not giving up. I am forever grateful for your listening ear, your partnership, and guidance in helping me achieve health.

To Cindy Perloff, you are the most amazing mentor and guide! My heart and life are full because you've shown me the way. Infinite love and gratitude.

Jeff Jimeson, thank you for seeing my potential and helping me rise to it. God knew exactly when to bring you into my life and I am so grateful for it!

"The essence of all beautiful art is gratitude." ~ Friedrich Nietzsche

About the Author

Angela Gaffney is the catalyst for healthy transformation. She works with executives and organizations that support the health of their employees and want to create an environment of personal and professional success.

It is possible to achieve health while fulfilling your personal and professional goals; Angela knows what it takes to make it happen. After surviving a health crisis that nearly took her life, she became a Certified Health Coach and has shared her proven strategies with hundreds of others.

Angela's presentations and workshops challenge attendees to think differently about their health. There's no crash diet, no need

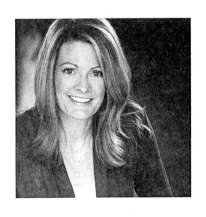

for intense willpower, or a restrictive lifestyle. Angela's simple strategies solve common health challenges, empower others to take charge of their health and ignite lifelong transformation.

Prior to starting Essential Health and Wellness, LLC, Angela worked for Johnson and Johnson in sales, training, and management and went on to serve the medical community as the Vice President of Sales and Business Development for Distance Learning Network. She relates well to the busy executive, traveling often and balancing the demands of work with quality family time.

Angela is a regular contributor to the *Huffington Post* and has published two cookbooks: *The Daily Essentials Cookbook Collection:*

Breakfast and *The Daily Essentials Cookbook Collection: Lunch.* She is a member of the National Speakers Association and regularly speaks and writes about wellness.

To hire Angela to speak at your next event, discuss a wellness program for your corporation, or take advantage of complimentary health tools, please visit www.AngelaGaffney.com.

Resources

Weil, MD, Andrew. "Stumped by Oxidative Stress?" *DrWeil.com*. Published March 17, 2009. Accessed July 31, 2016. http://www. drweil.com/drw/u/QAA400537/Stumped-by-Oxidative-Stress. html.

Websites:

Authority Nutrition
www.authoritynutrition.com

Centers for Disease Control
www.cdc.gov

Environmental Working Group
www.ewg.org

Mark Hyman, MD
www.drhyman.com

International Federation for Produce Standards
www.ifpsglobal.com

Institute for Integrative Nutrition
www.integrativenutrition.com

Food Marketing Institute
www.fmi.org

Gaia Yoga Resource
www.gaia.com

Dr. Joseph Mercola
www.mercola.com

The National Academies of Sciences, Engineering, Medicine
www.nationalacademies.org

The Non-GMO Project
www.nongmoproject.org

Andrew Weil, MD
www.drweil.com

The George Mateljan Foundation for The World's
Healthiest Foods
www.whfoods.com

Additional health resources and copies of the graphics found in this book are available to you at: www.AngelaGaffney.com.